The Definitive Guide to Mediterranean Meals

Amazing Recipes to Enjoy Your Meals and Boost Your Diet

Raymond Morton

Table of cotents

Masala Scallops..6

Cinnamon Tuna..8

Tuna and Kale...10

Lemongrass Mackerel...12

Scallops with Almonds.......................................14

Scallops and Leeks...16

Salmon and Broccoli Salad 18

Shrimp and Dates Salad....................................20

Salmon and Watercress Bowls.........................22

Trout and Butter Sauce......................................24

Kimchi Salmon 26

Salmon Meatballs and Sauce...........................28

Baked Lemon Haddock 31

Tilapia and Mayo Mix...33

Trout and Pecan Sauce..35

Salmon with Butter Caper Sauce.....................38

Grilled Oysters 40

Baked Butter Halibut..42

Herbed Tuna Cakes..44

Yogurt Cream 46

Strawberry Pudding...48

Coconut Bars...50

Cinnamon Apples..52

Coconut Cake..54

Cinnamon Cocoa Cake......................................56

Vanilla Cream 58
Blueberries Bowls 60
Brownies 62
Strawberries Coconut Cake 64
Cocoa Almond Pudding 66
Nutmeg Cream 68
Vanilla Avocado Cream 70
Raspberries Cream Cheese Bowls 72
Watermelon Salad 73
Coconut Apples 75
Orange Compote 77
Pears Stew 79
Lemon Watermelon Mix 81
Rhubarb Cream 83
Mango Bowls 84
Strawberry Stew 86
Lemon Pudding 88
Peach Cream 90
Vanilla Plums 91
Chia Apples 93
Rice Pudding 95
Almond Rhubarb Bowls 97
Lime Berry Cream 99
Mint Blueberries Bowls 101
Banana Cream 103
Muffins 105
Plums Bowls 107

Seed Bars 109

Masala Scallops

Prep time: 10 minutes I **Cooking time:** 20 minutes I
Servings: 4

Ingredients:

- 2 tablespoons olive oil
- 2 jalapenos, chopped
- 1 pound sea scallops
- A pinch of salt and black pepper
- ¼ teaspoon cinnamon powder
- 1 teaspoon garam masala
- 1 teaspoon coriander, ground
- 1 teaspoon cumin, ground
- 2 tablespoons cilantro, chopped

Directions:

1. Heat up a pan with the oil over medium heat, add the jalapenos, cinnamon and the other ingredients except the scallops and cook for 10 minutes.
2. Add the rest of the ingredients, toss, cook for 10 minutes more, divide into bowls and serve.

Nutrition info per serving: calories 251, fat 4, fiber 4, carbs 11, protein 17

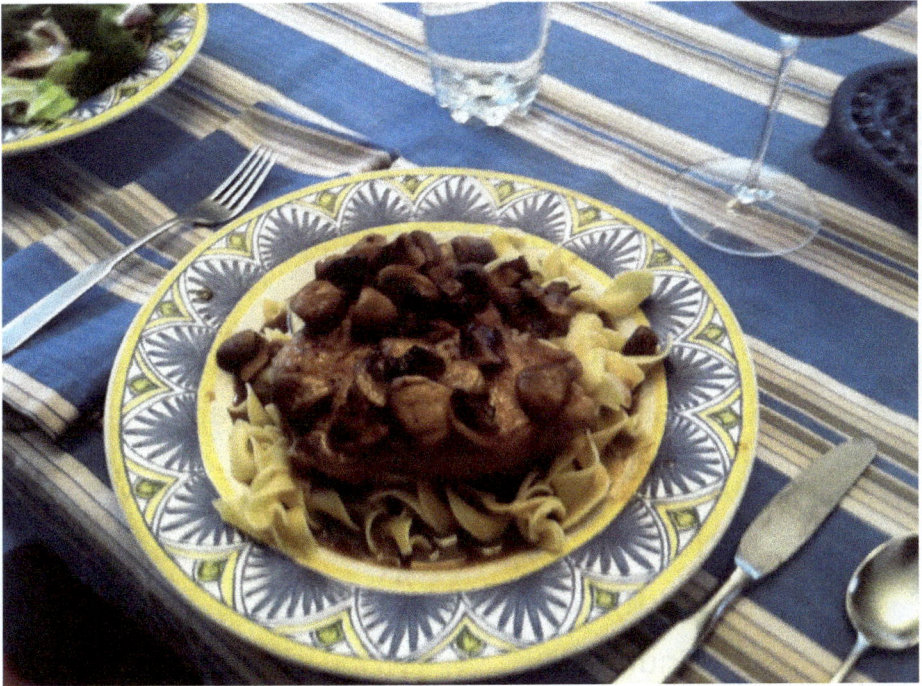

Cinnamon Tuna

Prep time: 5 minutes I **Cooking time:** 20 minutes I
Servings: 4

Ingredients:

- 1 yellow onion, chopped
- 1 tablespoon olive oil
- 1 pound tuna fillets, boneless, skinless and cubed
- 1 tablespoon cinnamon powder
- 1 red pepper, chopped
- 1 teaspoon sweet paprika
- 1 tablespoon coriander, chopped

Directions:

1. Heat up a pan with the oil over medium heat, add the onions and the pepper and cook for 5 minutes.
2. Add the fish and the other ingredients, cook everything for 15 minutes, divide between plates and serve.

Nutrition info per serving: calories 215, fat 4, fiber 7, carbs 14, protein 7

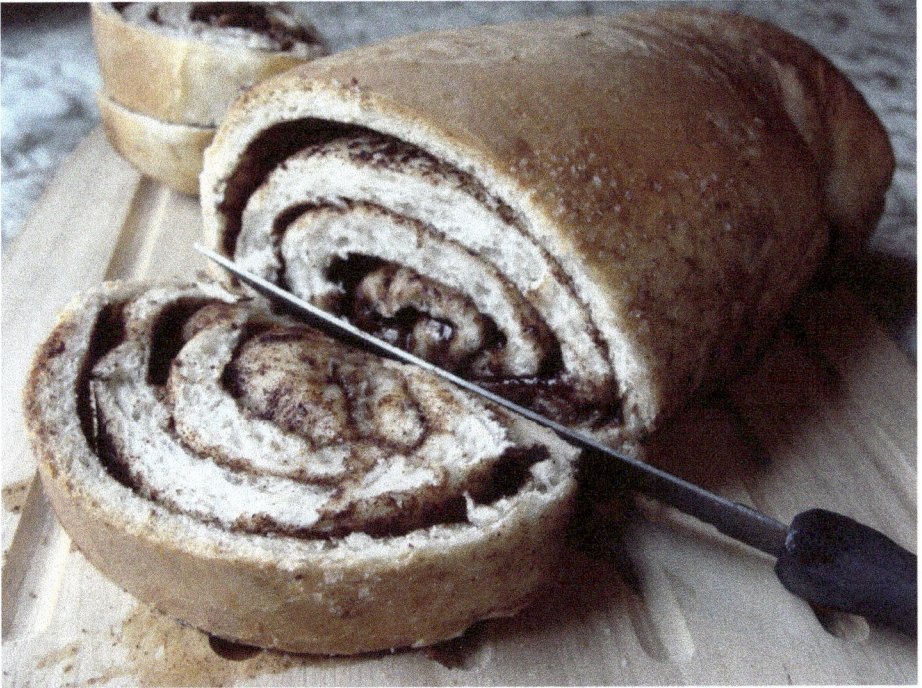

Tuna and Kale

Prep time: 5 minutes I **Cooking time:** 20 minutes I
Servings: 4

Ingredients:

- 1 pound tuna fillets, boneless, skinless and cubed
- A pinch of salt and black pepper
- 2 tablespoons olive oil
- 1 cup kale, torn
- ½ cup cherry tomatoes, cubed
- 1 yellow onion, chopped

Directions:

1. Heat up a pan with the oil over medium heat, add the onion and sauté for 5 minutes.
2. Add the tuna and the other ingredients, toss, cook everything for 15 minutes more, divide between plates and serve.

Nutrition info per serving: calories 251, fat 4, fiber 7, carbs 14, protein 7

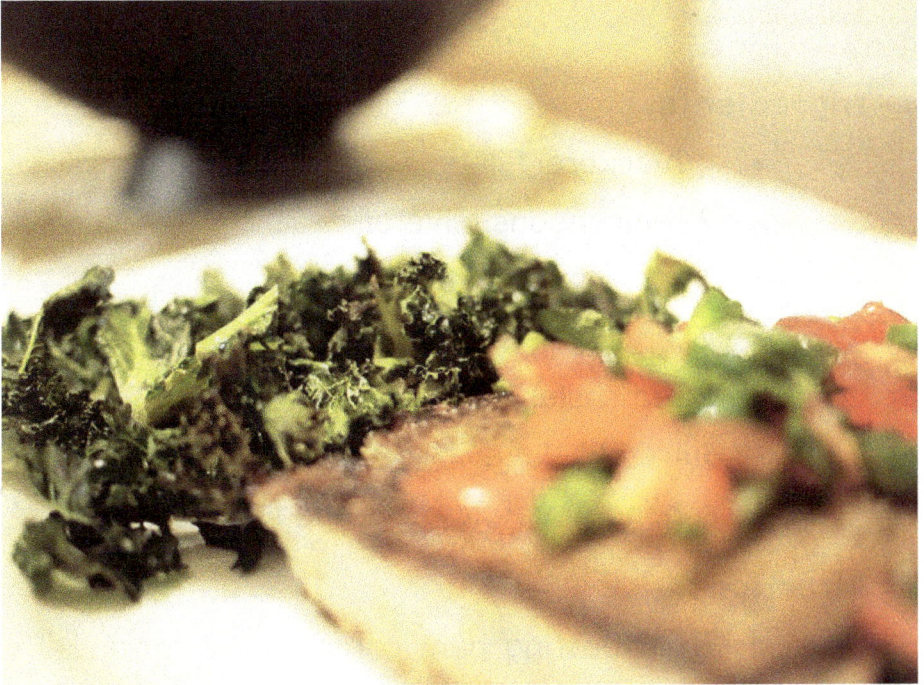

Lemongrass Mackerel

Prep time: 10 minutes I **Cooking time:** 25 minutes I
Servings: 4

Ingredients:

- 4 mackerel fillets, skinless and boneless
- 2 tablespoons olive oil
- 1 tablespoon ginger, grated
- 2 lemongrass sticks, chopped
- 2 red chilies, chopped
- Juice of 1 lime
- A handful parsley, chopped

Directions:

1. In a roasting pan, combine the mackerel with the oil, ginger and the other ingredients, toss and bake at 390 degrees F for 25 minutes.
2. Divide everything between plates and serve.

Nutrition info per serving: calories 251, fat 3, fiber 4, carbs 14, protein 8

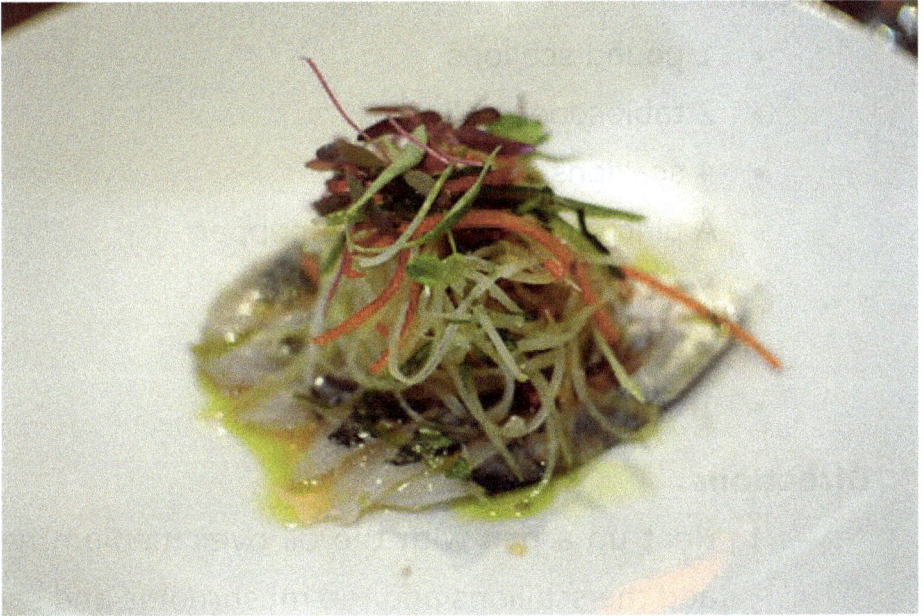

Scallops with Almonds

Prep time: 5 minutes I **Cooking time:** 10 minutes I
Servings: 4

Ingredients:

- 1 pound scallops
- 2 tablespoons olive oil
- 4 scallions, chopped
- A pinch of salt and black pepper
- ½ cup mushrooms, sliced
- 2 tablespoon almonds, chopped
- 1 cup coconut cream

Directions:

1. Heat up a pan with the oil over medium heat, add the scallions and the mushrooms and sauté for 2 minutes.
2. Add the scallops and the other ingredients, toss, cook over medium heat for 8 minutes more, divide into bowls and serve.

Nutrition info per serving: calories 322, fat 23.7, fiber 2.2, carbs 8.1, protein 21.6

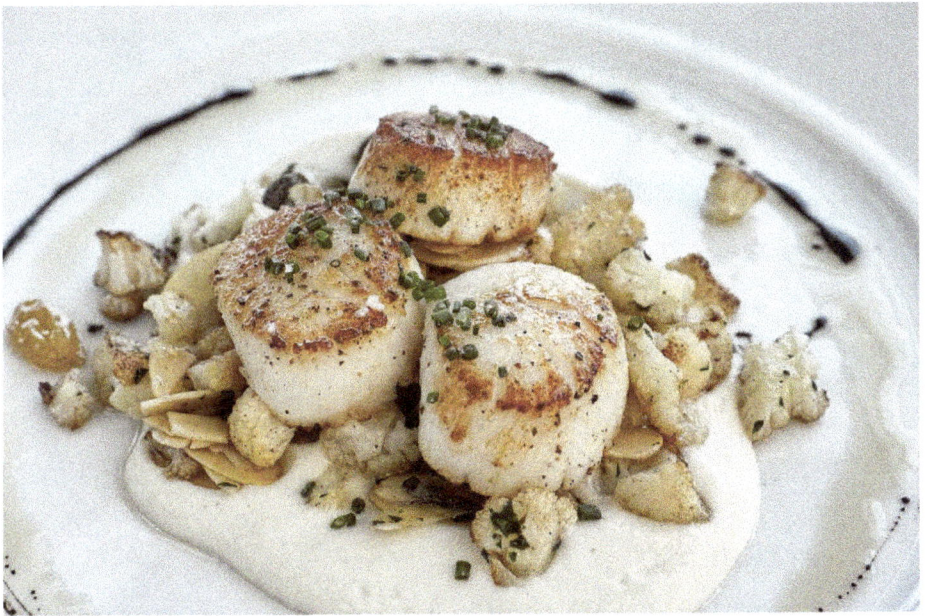

Scallops and Leeks

Prep time: 5 minutes I **Cooking time:** 22 minutes I
Servings: 4

Ingredients:

- 1 pound scallops
- ½ teaspoon rosemary, dried
- ½ teaspoon oregano, dried
- 2 tablespoons avocado oil
- 1 yellow onion, chopped
- 2 leeks, sliced
- ½ cup chicken stock
- 1 tablespoon cilantro, chopped
- A pinch of salt and black pepper

Directions:

1. Heat up a pan with the oil over medium heat, add the onion and sauté for 2 minutes.
2. Add the leeks and the stock, toss and cook for 10 minutes more.
3. Add the scallops and the remaining ingredients, toss, cook for another 10 minutes, divide everything into bowls and serve.

Nutrition info per serving: calories 211, fat 2, fiber 4.1, carbs 26.9, protein 20.7

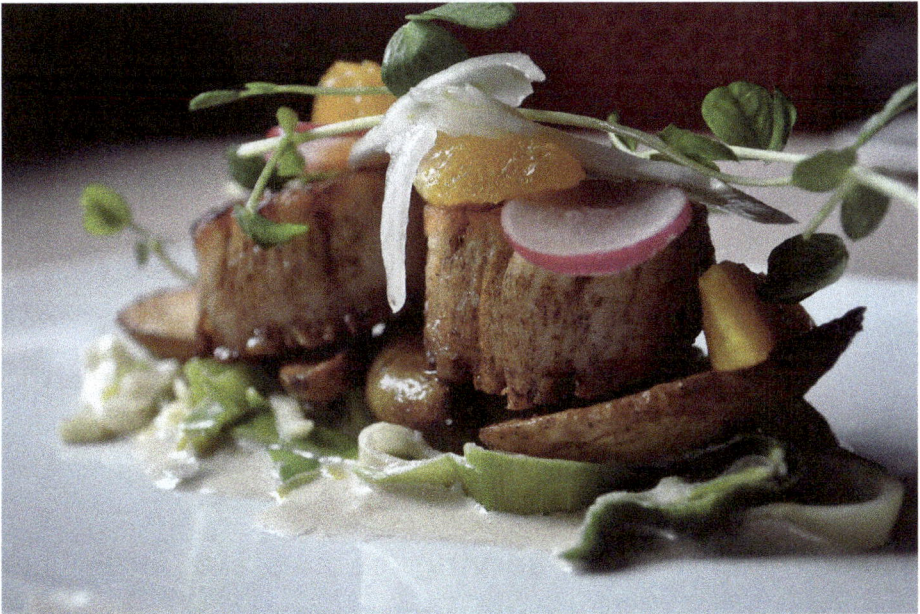

Salmon and Broccoli Salad

Prep time: 5 minutes I **Cooking time:** 0 minutes I
Servings: 4

Ingredients:

- 1 cup smoked salmon, boneless and flaked
- 1 cup broccoli florets, cooked
- ½ cup baby arugula
- 1 tablespoon lemon juice
- 2 spring onions, chopped
- 1 tablespoon olive oil
- A pinch of sea salt and black pepper

Directions:

1. In a salad bowl, combine the salmon with the broccoli and the other ingredients, toss and serve.

Nutrition info per serving: calories 210, fat 6, fiber 5, carbs 10, protein 12

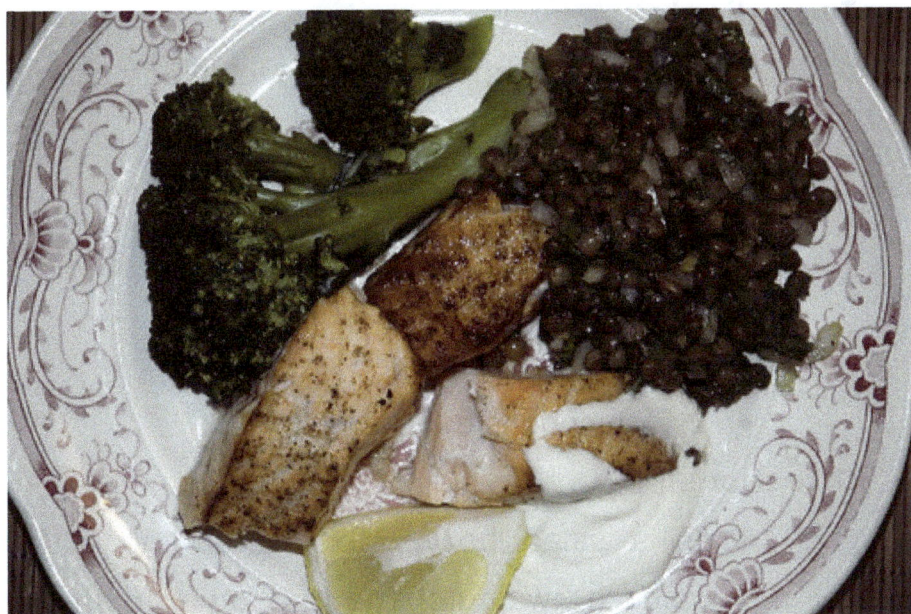

Shrimp and Dates Salad

Prep time: 10 minutes I **Cooking time:** 0 minutes I
Servings: 4

Ingredients:

- 1 pound shrimp, cooked, peeled and deveined
- 2 cups baby spinach
- 2 tablespoons walnuts, chopped
- 1 cup cherry tomatoes, halved
- 1 tablespoon lemon juice
- ½ cup dates, chopped
- 2 tablespoons avocado oil

Directions:

1. In a salad bowl, mix the shrimp with the spinach, walnuts and the other ingredients, toss and serve.

Nutrition info per serving: calories 243, fat 5.4, fiber 3.3, carbs 21.6, protein 28.3

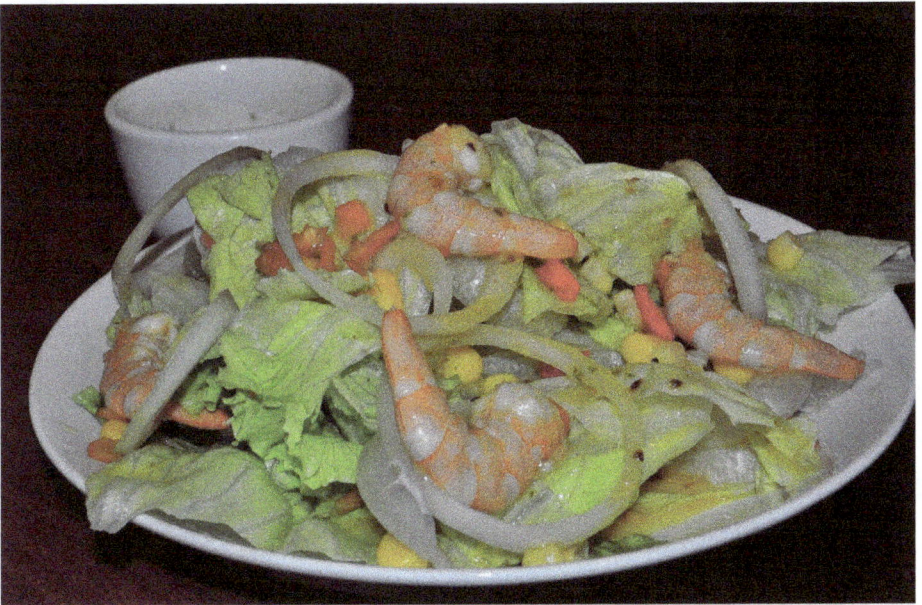

Salmon and Watercress Bowls

Prep time: 10 minutes I **Cooking time:** 0 minutes I
Servings: 4

Ingredients:

- 1 pound smoked salmon, boneless, skinless and flaked
- 2 spring onions, chopped
- 2 tablespoons avocado oil
- ½ cup baby arugula
- 1 cup watercress
- 1 tablespoon lemon juice
- 1 cucumber, sliced
- 1 avocado, peeled, pitted and roughly cubed
- A pinch of sea salt and black pepper

Directions:

1. In a salad bowl, mix the salmon with the spring onions, watercress and the other ingredients, toss and serve.

Nutrition info per serving: calories 261, fat 15.8, fiber 4.4, carbs 8.2, protein 22.7

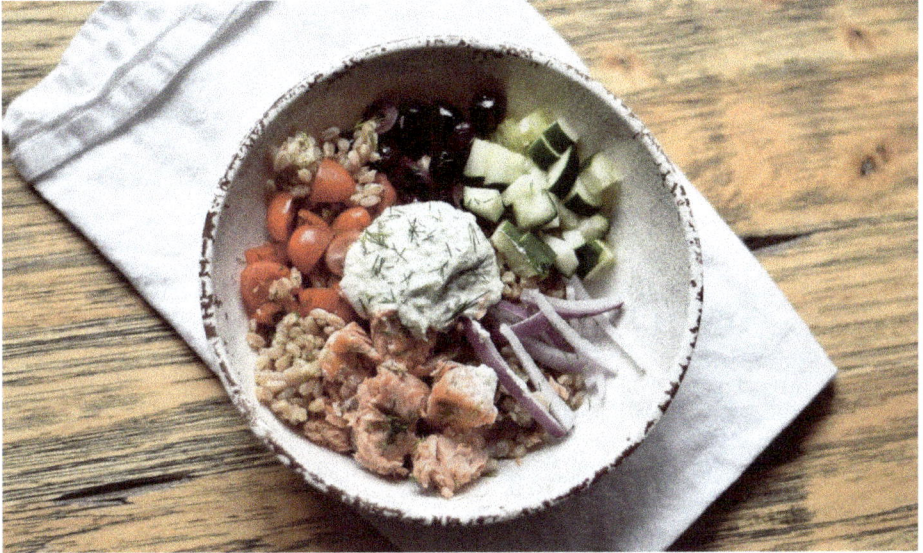

Trout and Butter Sauce

Prep time: 10 minutes I **Cooking time:** 10 minutes I
Servings: 4

Ingredients:

- 4 trout fillets
- Salt and ground black pepper, to taste
- 3 teaspoons lemon zest, grated
- 3 tablespoons fresh chives, chopped
- 6 tablespoons butter
- 2 tablespoons olive oil
- 2 teaspoons lemon juice

Directions:

1. Season trout with salt, pepper, drizzle olive oil, and massage into fish.
2. Heat a kitchen grill over medium–high heat, add fish fillets, cook for 4 minutes, flip, and cook for 4 minutes.
3. Heat a pan with the butter over medium heat, add salt, pepper, chives, lemon juice, lemon zest, and stir well.

4. Divide fish fillets on plates, drizzle the butter sauce over them, and serve.

Nutrition info per serving: Calories – 333, Fat – 29.6, Fiber – 0.2, Carbs – 0.5, Protein – 16.8

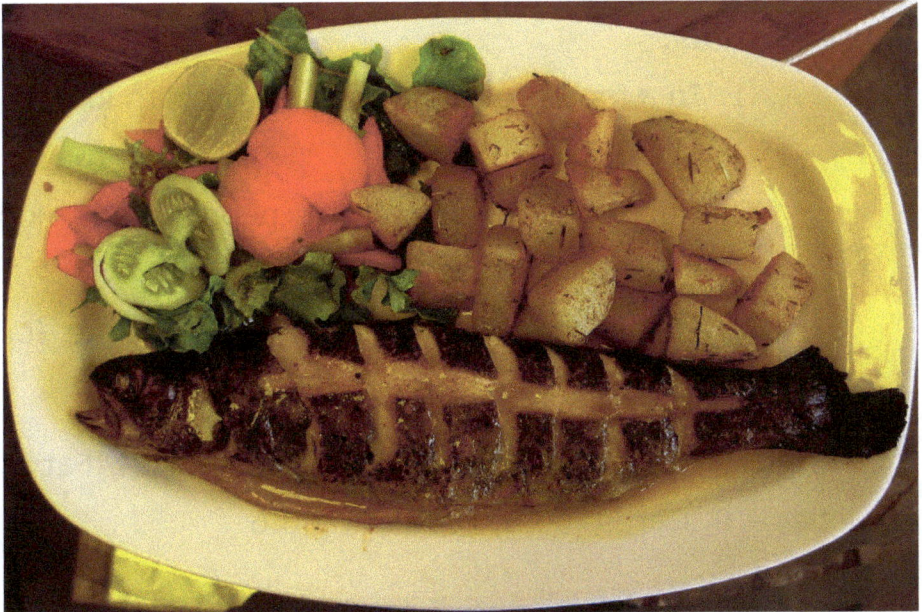

Kimchi Salmon

Prep time: 10 minutes I **Cooking time:** 12 minutes I **Servings:** 4

Ingredients:

- 2 tablespoons butter, softened
- 1¼ pound salmon fillet
- 2 ounces kimchi, diced
- Salt and ground black pepper, to taste

Directions:

1. In a food processor, mix butter with kimchi and blend well.
2. Rub salmon with salt, pepper, and kimchi mixture, and place into a baking dish.
3. Place in an oven at 425ºF and bake for 15 minutes. Divide on plates and serve.

Nutrition info per serving: Calories – 467, Fat – 25, Fiber – 0, Carbs – 0.5, Protein – 60.6

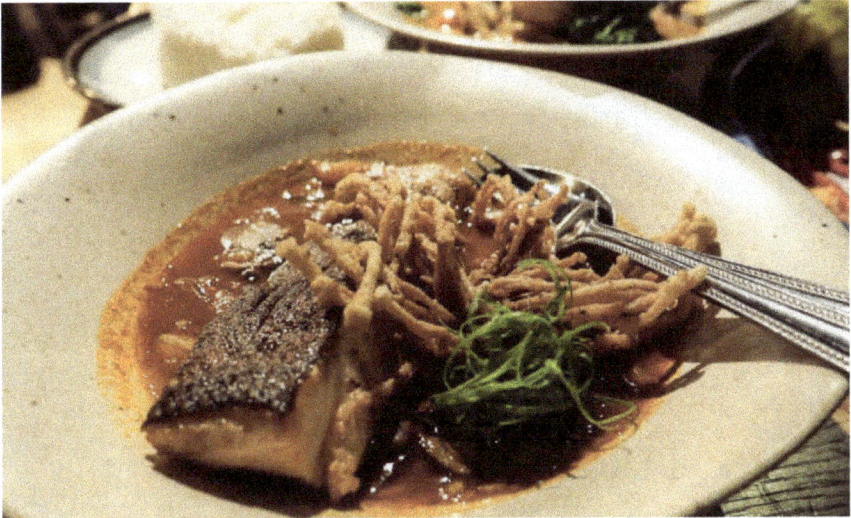

Salmon Meatballs and Sauce

Prep time: 10 minutes I **Cooking time:** 30 minutes I
Servings: 4

Ingredients:

- 2 tablespoons butter
- 2 garlic cloves, peeled and minced
- ⅓ cup onion, peeled and chopped
- 1 pound wild salmon, boneless and minced
- ¼ cup fresh chives, chopped
- 1 egg
- 2 tablespoons Dijon mustard
- 1 tablespoon coconut flour
- Salt and ground black pepper, to taste

For the sauce:

- 4 garlic cloves, peeled and minced
- 2 tablespoons butter
- 2 tablespoons Dijon mustard
- Juice, and zest of 1 lemon
- 2 cups coconut cream
- 2 tablespoons fresh chives, chopped

Directions:

1. Heat a pan with 2 tablespoons butter over medium heat, add onion and 2 garlic cloves, stir, cook for 3 minutes, and transfer to a bowl.
2. In another bowl, mix the onion and garlic with salmon, chives, coconut flour, salt, pepper, 2 tablespoons mustard, egg, and stir well.
3. Shape meatballs from salmon mixture, place on a baking sheet, place in an oven at 350ºF, and bake for 25 minutes.
4. Heat a pan with 2 tablespoons butter over medium heat, add 4 garlic cloves, stir, and cook for 1 minute.
5. Add coconut cream, 2 tablespoons Dijon mustard, lemon juice, lemon zest, chives, stir, and cook for 3 minutes.
6. Take salmon meatballs out of the oven, drop them into the Dijon sauce, toss, cook for 1 minute, and take off the heat. Divide into bowls and serve.

Nutrition info per serving: Calories – 575, Fat – 47.1, Fiber – 3.4, Carbs – 9, Protein – 31.9

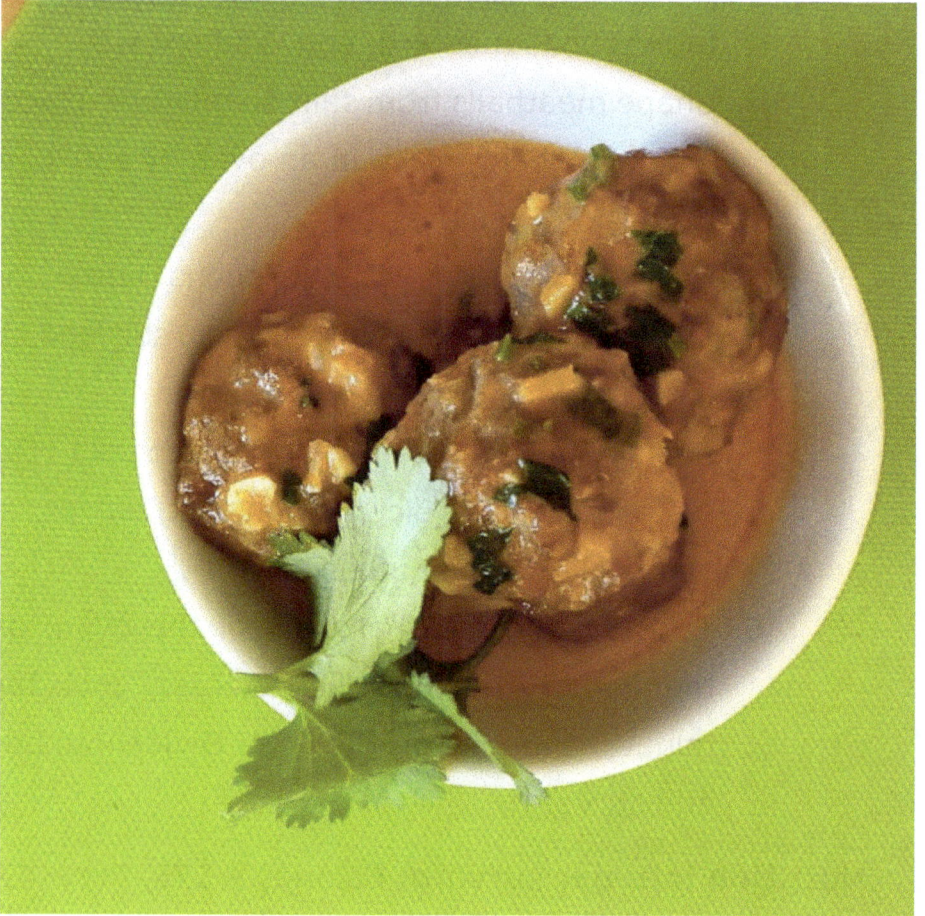

Baked Lemon Haddock

Prep time: 10 minutes I **Cooking time:** 30 minutes I
Servings: 4

Ingredients:

- 1 pound haddock
- 3 teaspoons water
- 2 tablespoons lemon juice
- Salt and ground black pepper, to taste
- 2 tablespoons mayonnaise
- 1 teaspoon dill weed
- Vegetable oil cooking spray
- A pinch of Old Bay Seasoning

Directions:

1. Spray a baking dish with some cooking oil.
2. Add lemon juice, water, fish, and toss to coat. Add salt, pepper, Old Bay Seasoning, dill, and toss again. Add mayonnaise and spread well.
3. Place in an oven at 350ºF, and bake for 30 minutes. Divide on plates and serve.

Nutrition info per serving: Calories – 121, Fat – 3.5, Fiber – 0, Carbs – 1.9, Protein –20.1

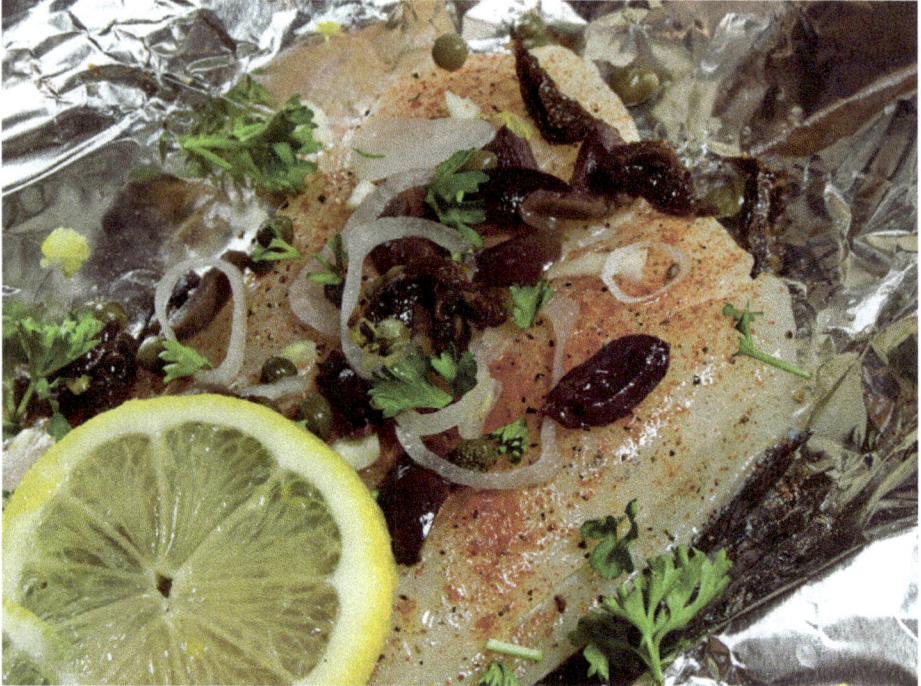

Tilapia and Mayo Mix

Prep time: 10 minutes I **Cooking time:** 10 minutes I
Servings: 4

Ingredients:

- 4 tilapia fillets, boneless
- Salt and ground black pepper, to taste
- ½ cup Parmesan cheese, grated
- 4 tablespoons mayonnaise
- ¼ teaspoon dried basil
- ¼ teaspoon garlic powder
- 2 tablespoons lemon juice
- ¼ cup butter
- Vegetable oil cooking spray
- A pinch of onion powder

Directions:

1. Spray a baking sheet with cooking spray, and arrange the tilapia on the tray.
2. Season with salt, pepper, place under a preheated broiler, and cook for 3 minutes.
3. Turn the fish and broil for 3 minutes.
4. In a bowl, mix Parmesan cheese with mayonnaise, basil, garlic, lemon juice, onion powder, butter, and stir well.
5. Add fish to mixture, toss to coat well, place on baking sheet again, and broil for 3 minutes. Transfer to plates and serve.

Nutrition info per serving: calories 300, fat 20.5, fiber 0.1, carbs 4.3, protein 25.9

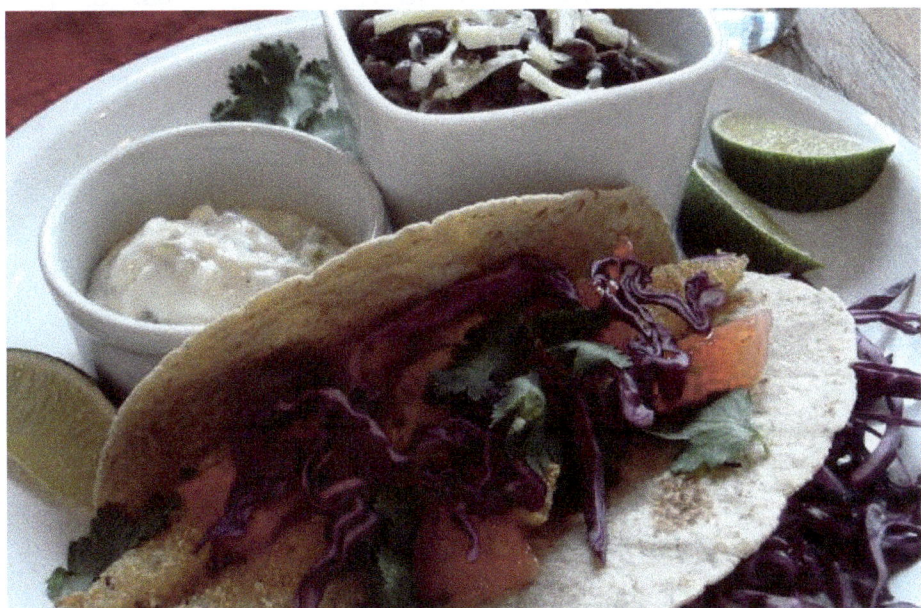

Trout and Pecan Sauce

Prep time: 10 minutes I **Cooking time:** 10 minutes I **Servings:** 1

Ingredients:

- 1 trout fillet
- Salt and ground black pepper, to taste
- 1 tablespoon olive oil
- 1 tablespoon butter
- Zest, and juice from 1 lemon
- ½ cup fresh parsley, chopped
- ½ cup pecans, chopped

Directions:

1. Heat a pan with the oil over medium–high heat, add fish fillet, season with salt, pepper, cook for 4 minutes on each side, transfer to a plate and keep warm.
2. Heat the same pan with butter over medium heat, add pecans, stir, and toast for 1 minutes.
3. Add lemon juice, lemon zest, some salt, pepper, and chopped parsley, stir, cook for 1 minute, and pour over the fish fillets, and serve.

Nutrition info per serving: calories 838, fat 81, fiber 8.5, carbs 11.9, protein 25

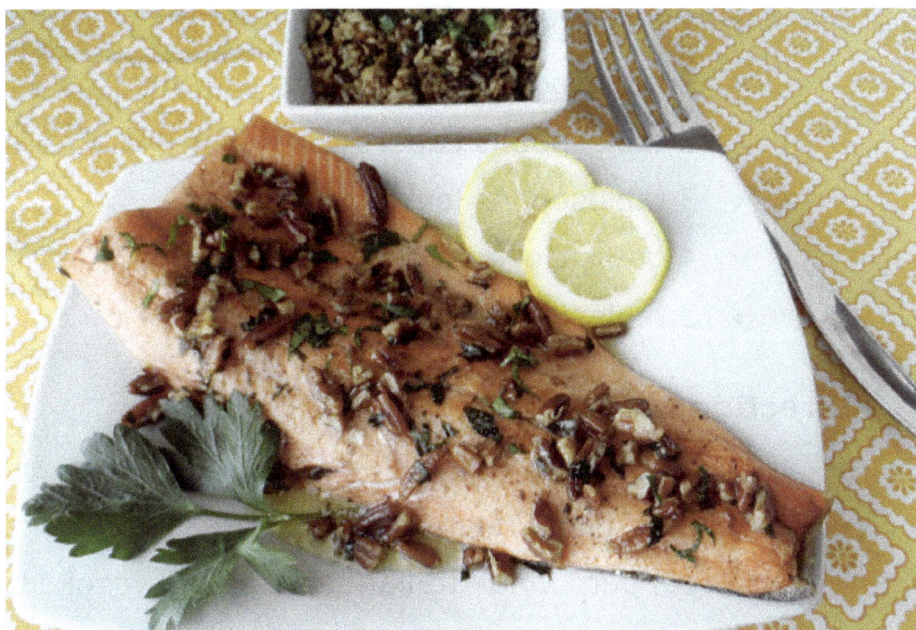

Salmon with Butter Caper Sauce

Prep time: 10 minutes I **Cooking time:** 20 minutes I
Servings: 3

Ingredients:

- 3 salmon fillets
- Salt and ground black pepper, to taste
- 1 tablespoon olive oil
- 1 tablespoon Italian seasoning
- 2 tablespoons capers
- 3 tablespoons lemon juice
- 4 garlic cloves, peeled and minced
- 2 tablespoons butter

Directions:

1. Heat a pan with olive oil over medium heat, add fish fillets skin side up, season with salt, pepper, and Italian seasoning, cook for 2 minutes, flip, and cook for 2 minutes, take off heat, cover pan, and set aside for 15 minutes.
2. Transfer fish to a plate, and leave them aside.
3. Heat the same pan over medium heat, add capers, lemon juice, and garlic, stir, and cook for 2 minutes.

4. Take pan off the heat, add the butter, and stir well.

5. Return fish to pan, and toss to coat with the sauce. Divide on plates and serve.

Nutrition info per serving: Calories – 369, Fat – 24.9, Fiber – 0.3, Carbs – 2.4, Protein – 35.

1

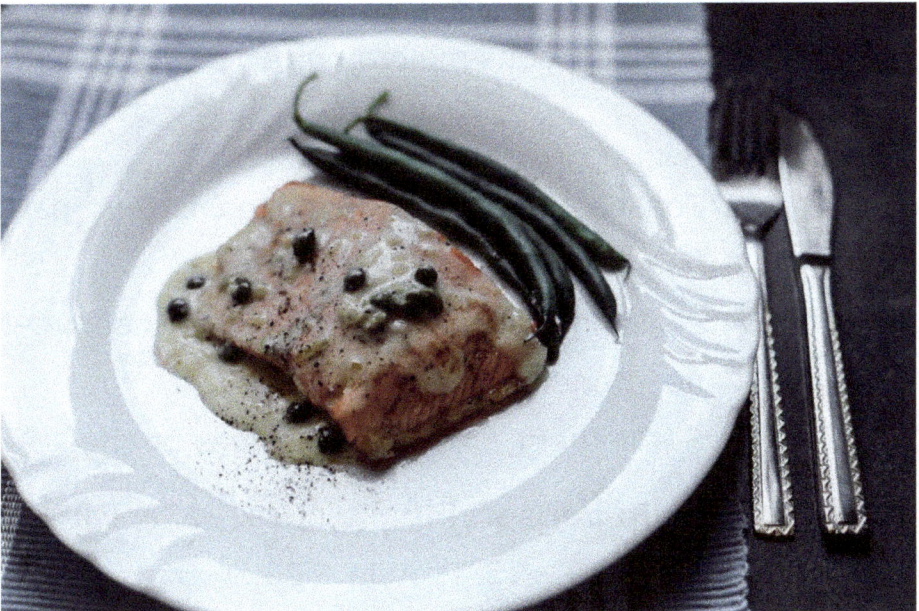

Grilled Oysters

Prep time: 10 minutes I **Cooking time:** 10 minutes I
Servings: 3

Ingredients:

- 6 oysters, shucked
- 3 garlic cloves, peeled and minced
- 1 lemon, cut in wedges
- 1 tablespoon parsley
- A pinch of sweet paprika
- 2 tablespoons melted butter

Directions:

1. Top each oyster with melted butter, parsley, paprika, and butter.
2. Place on preheated grill pan over medium–high heat, and cook for 8 minutes.
3. Serve them with lemon wedges on the side.

Nutrition info per serving: Calories – 272, Fat – 15.7, Fiber – 0.1, Carbs – 13, Protein – 20.3

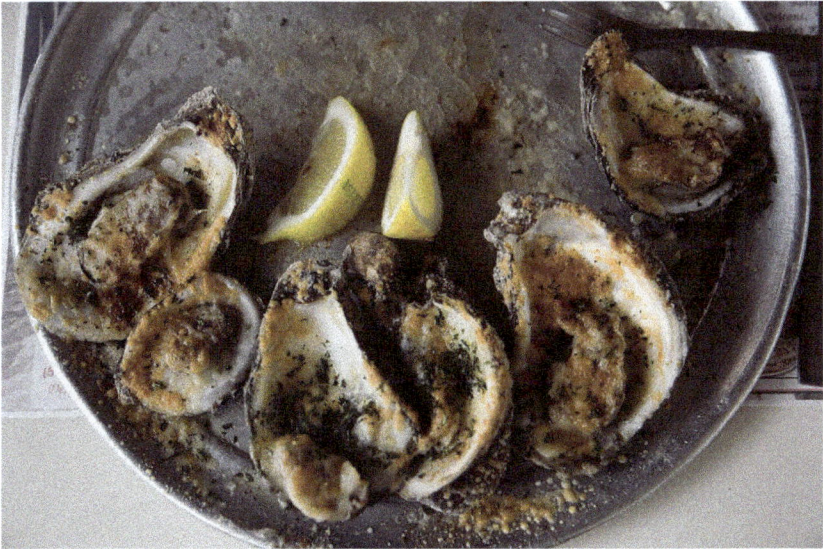

Baked Butter Halibut

Prep time: 10 minutes I **Cooking time:** 10 minutes I
Servings: 4

Ingredients:

- ½ cup Parmesan cheese, grated
- ¼ cup butter
- 2 tablespoons green onions, chopped
- 6 garlic cloves, peeled and minced
- A dash of Tabasco sauce
- 4 halibut fillets, boneless
- Salt and ground black pepper, to taste
- Juice of ½ lemon

Directions:

1. Season halibut with salt, pepper, and some of the lemon juice, place in a baking dish, and cook in the oven at 450ºF for 6 minutes.
2. Heat a pan with butter over medium heat, add Parmesan cheese, mayonnaise, green onions, Tabasco sauce, garlic, remaining lemon juice, and stir well.

3. Take fish out of the oven, drizzle cheese sauce all over, turn the oven to broil, and broil the fish for 3 minutes. Divide on plates and serve.

Nutrition info per serving: Calories – 530, Fat – 26.2, Fiber – 0.2, Carbs – 5.7, Protein – 65.6

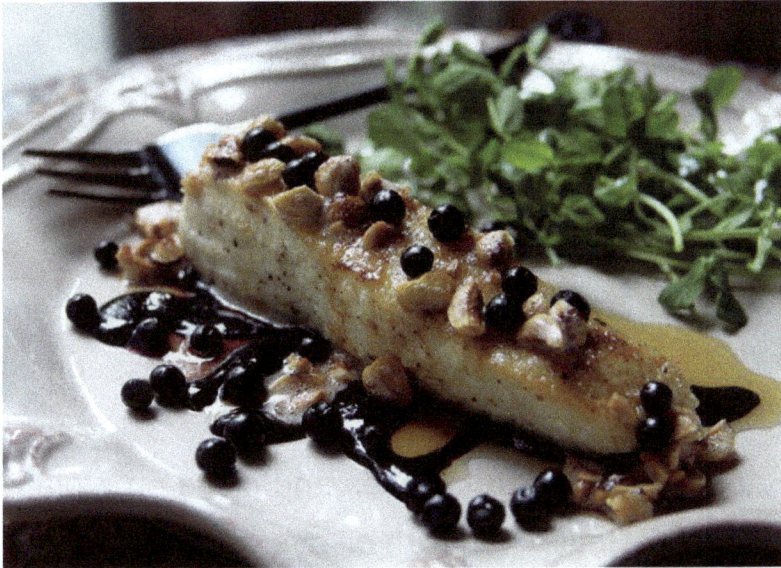

Herbed Tuna Cakes

Prep time: 10 minutes I **Cooking time:** 10 minutes I
Servings: 12

Ingredients:

- 15 ounces smoked tuna, flaked
- 3 eggs
- ½ teaspoon dried dill
- 1 teaspoon dried parsley
- ½ cup onion chopped
- 1 teaspoon garlic powder
- Salt and ground black pepper, to taste
- Oil, for frying

Directions:

1. In a bowl, mix tuna with salt, pepper, dill, parsley, onion, garlic powder, eggs, and stir well.
2. Shape tuna cakes and place on a plate.
3. Heat a pan with oil over medium–high heat, add tuna cakes, cook for 5 minutes on each side. Divide on plates and serve.

Nutrition info per serving: Calories – 84, Fat – 4, Fiber – 0.1, Carbs – 0.6, Protein – 10.8

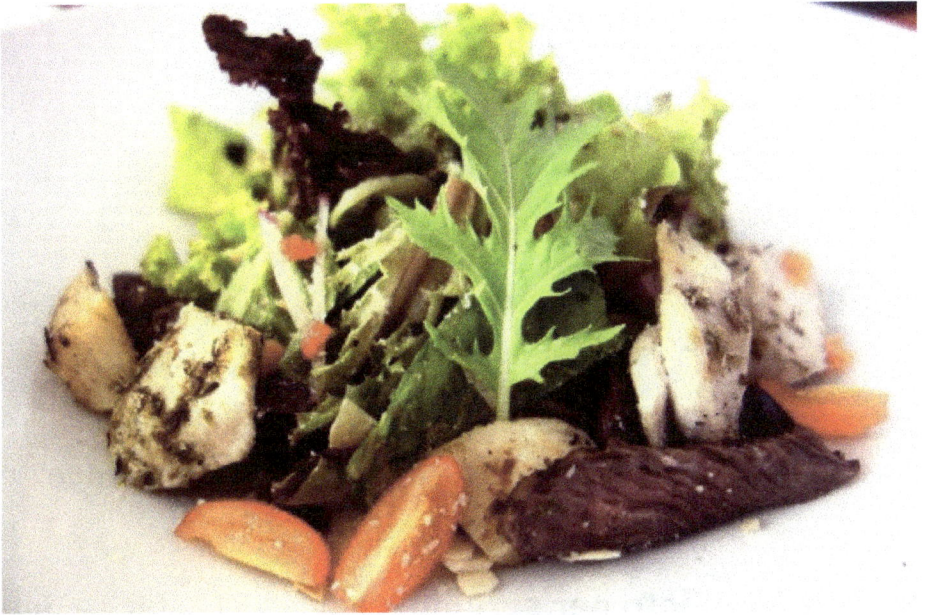

Yogurt Cream

Prep time: 2 hours and 4 minutes I **Cooking time:** 0 minutes I **Servings:** 4

Ingredients:

- 4 cups Greek yogurt
- 1 cup coconut cream
- 3 tablespoons stevia
- 2 teaspoons lime zest, grated
- 1 tablespoon mint, chopped

Directions:

1. In a blender, combine the cream with the yogurt and the other ingredients, pulse well, divide into cups and keep in the fridge for 2 hours before serving.

Nutrition info per serving: calories 512, fat 14.3, fiber 1.5, carbs 83.6, protein 12.1

47

Strawberry Pudding

Prep time: 10 minutes I **Cooking time:** 24 minutes I
Servings: 4

Ingredients:

- 1 cup raspberries
- 2 teaspoons coconut sugar
- 3 eggs, whisked
- 1 tablespoon avocado oil
- ½ cup almond milk
- ½ cup coconut flour
- ¼ cup non-fat yogurt

Directions:

1. In a bowl, combine the raspberries with the sugar and the other ingredients except the cooking spray and whisk well.
2. Grease a pudding pan with the cooking spray, add the raspberries mix, spread, bake in the oven at 400 degrees F for 24 minutes, divide between dessert plates and serve.

Nutrition info per serving: calories 215, fat 11.3, fiber 3.4, carbs 21.3, protein 6.7

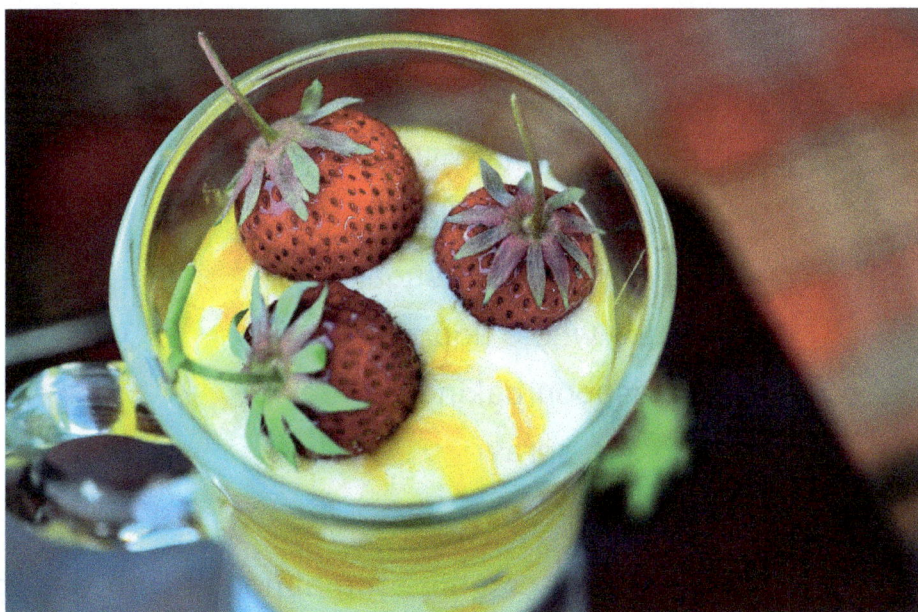

Coconut Bars

Prep time: 10 minutes I **Cooking time:** 30 minutes I
Servings: 4

Ingredients:

- 1 cup almonds, crushed
- 2 eggs, whisked
- ½ cup almond milk
- 1 teaspoon vanilla extract
- 2/3 cup coconut sugar
- 2 cups whole flour
- 1 teaspoon baking powder
- Cooking spray

Directions:

1. In a bowl, combine the almonds with the eggs and the other ingredients except the cooking spray and stir well.
2. Pour this into a square pan greased with cooking spray, spread well, bake in the oven for 30 minutes, cool down, cut into bars and serve.

Nutrition info per serving: calories 463, fat 22.5, fiber 11, carbs 54.4, protein 16.9

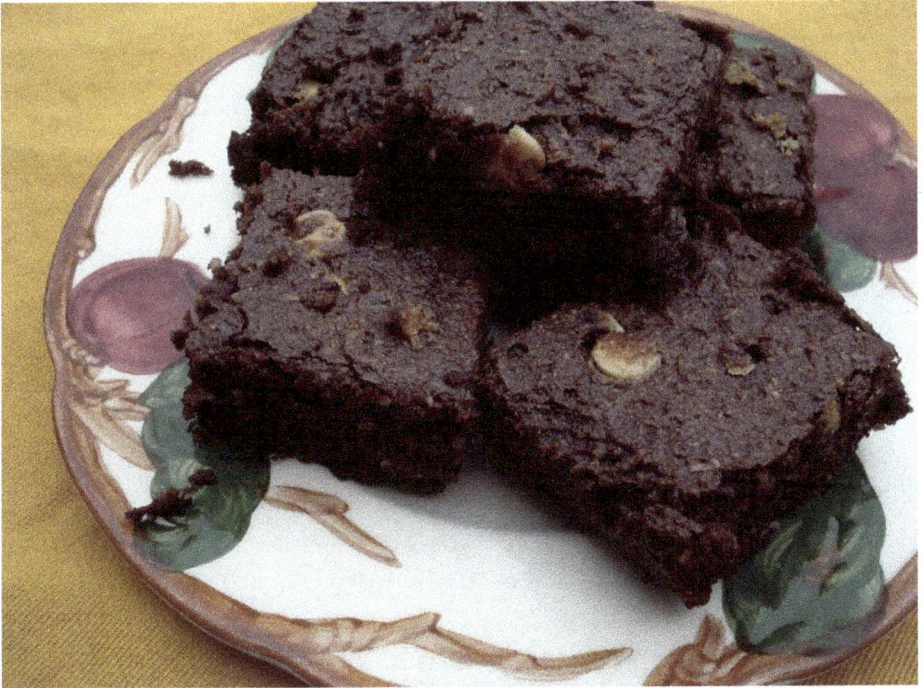

Cinnamon Apples

Prep time: 10 minutes I **Cooking time:** 30 minutes I
Servings: 4

Ingredients:

- 4 peaches, stones removed and halved
- 1 tablespoon coconut sugar
- 1 teaspoon vanilla extract
- ¼ teaspoon cinnamon powder
- 1 tablespoon avocado oil

Directions:

1. In a baking pan, combine the peaches with the sugar and the other ingredients, bake at 375 degrees F for 30 minutes, cool down and serve.

Nutrition info per serving: calories 91, fat 0.8, fiber 2.5, carb 19.2, protein 1.7

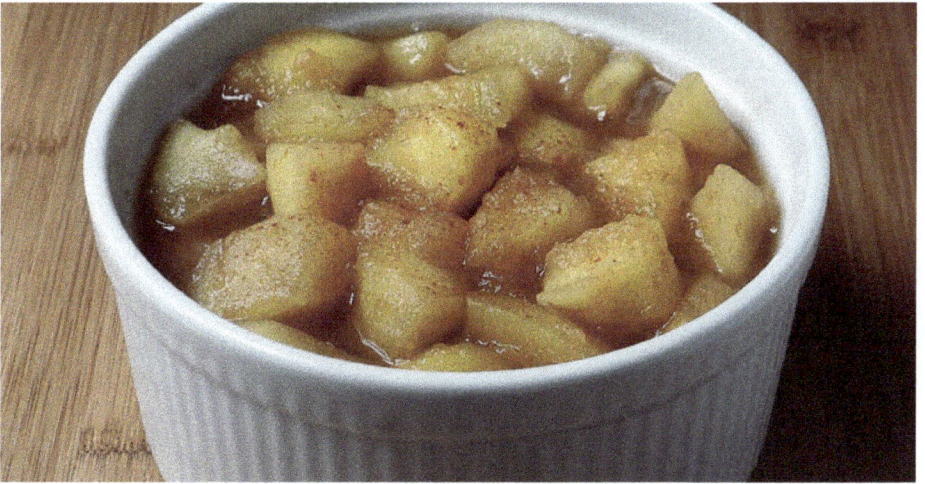

Coconut Cake

Prep time: 10 minutes I **Cooking time:** 25 minutes I
Servings: 8

Ingredients:

- 3 cups almond flour
- 1 cup coconut sugar
- 1 tablespoon vanilla extract
- ½ cup walnuts, chopped
- 2 teaspoons baking soda
- 2 cups coconut milk
- ½ cup coconut oil, melted

Directions:

1. In a bowl, combine the almond flour with the sugar and the other ingredients, whisk well, pour into a cake pan, spread, introduce in the oven at 370 degrees F, bake for 25 minutes.
2. Leave the cake to cool down, slice and serve.

Nutrition info per serving: calories 445, fat 10, fiber 6.5, carbs 31.4, protein 23.5

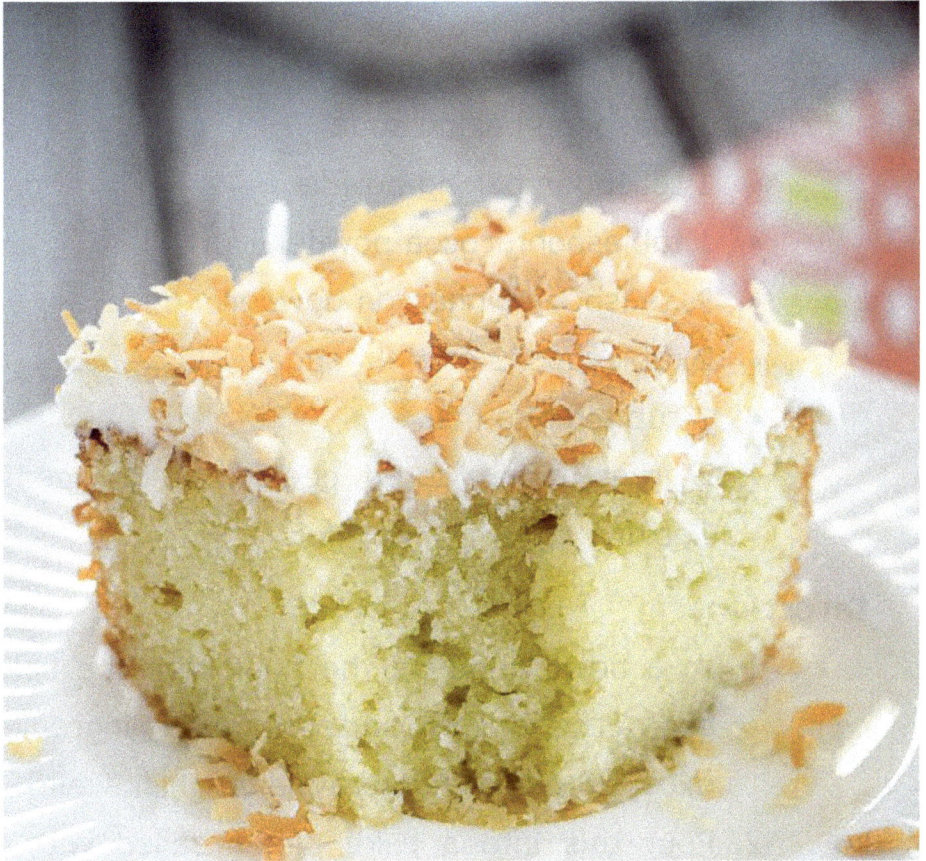

Cinnamon Cocoa Cake

Prep time: 10 minutes I **Cooking time:** 30 minutes I
Servings: 4

Ingredients:

- 2 cups almond flour
- 1 teaspoon baking soda
- 1 teaspoon baking powder
- 1 tablespoon cocoa powder
- ½ teaspoon cinnamon powder
- 2 tablespoons coconut sugar
- 1 cup almond milk
- 2 green apples, cored, peeled and chopped
- Cooking spray

Directions:

1. In a bowl, combine the flour with the baking soda, the apples and the other ingredients except the cooking spray, and whisk well.
2. Pour this into a cake pan greased with the cooking spray, spread well, introduce in the oven and bake at 360 degrees F for 30 minutes.
3. Cool the cake down, slice and serve.

Nutrition info per serving: calories 332, fat 22.4, fiber 9l.6, carbs 22.2, protein 12.3

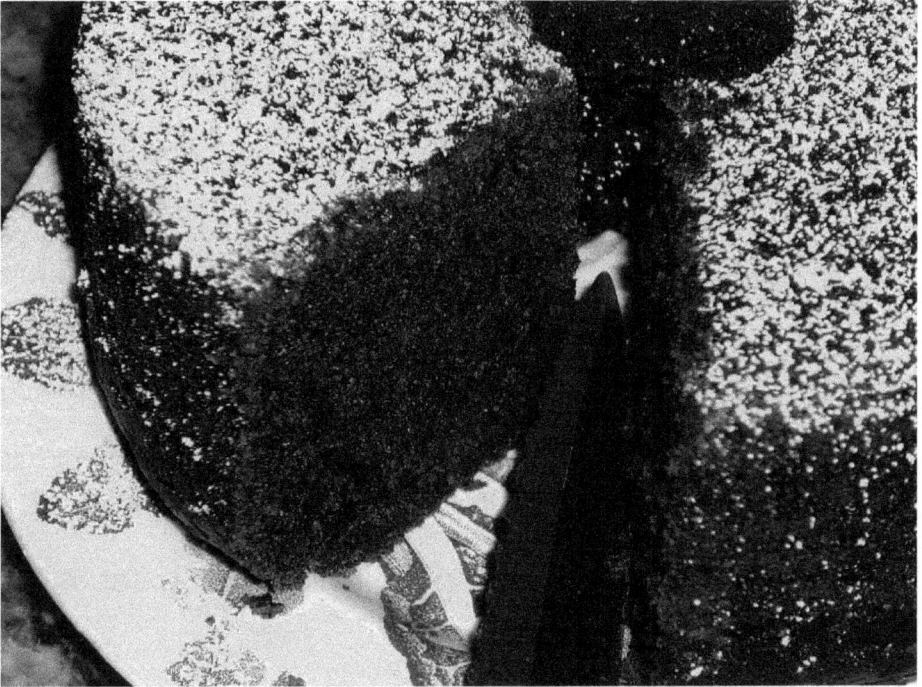

Vanilla Cream

Prep time: 2 hours I **Cooking time:** 10 minutes I
Servings: 4

Ingredients:

- 1 cup almond milk
- 1 cup coconut cream
- 2 cups coconut sugar
- 2 tablespoons cinnamon powder
- 1 teaspoon vanilla extract

Directions:

1. Heat up a pan with the almond milk over medium heat, add the rest of the ingredients, whisk, and cook for 10 minutes more.
2. Divide the mix into bowls, cool down and keep in the fridge for 2 hours before serving.

Nutrition info per serving: calories 254, fat 7.5, fiber 5, carbs 16.4, protein 9.5

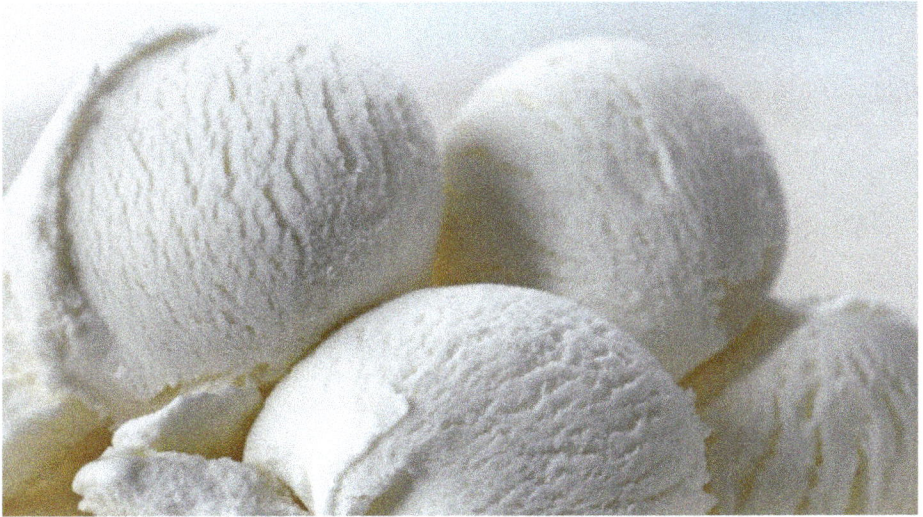

Blueberries Bowls

Prep time: 10 minutes I **Cooking time:** 0 minutes I
Servings: 4

Ingredients:

- 1 teaspoon vanilla extract
- 2 cups blueberries
- 1 teaspoon coconut sugar
- 8 ounces Greek yogurt

Directions:

1. In a bowl, combine the strawberries with the vanilla and the other ingredients, toss and serve cold.

Nutrition info per serving: calories 343, fat 13.4, fiber 6, carb 15.43, protein 5.5

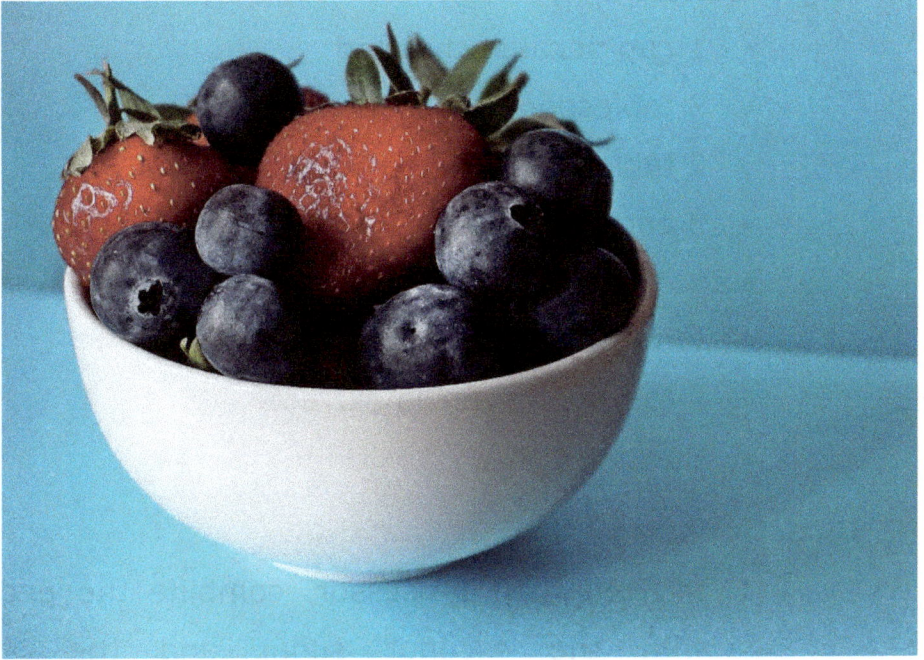

Brownies

Prep time: 10 minutes I **Cooking time:** 25 minutes I
Servings: 8

Ingredients:

- 1 cup pecans, chopped
- 3 tablespoons coconut sugar
- 2 tablespoons cocoa powder
- 3 eggs, whisked
- ¼ cup avocado oil
- ½ teaspoon baking powder
- 2 teaspoons vanilla extract
- Cooking spray

Directions:

1. In your food processor, combine the pecans with the coconut sugar and the other ingredients except the cooking spray and pulse well.
2. Grease a square pan with cooking spray, add the brownies mix, spread, introduce in the oven, bake at 350 degrees F for 25 minutes, leave aside to cool down, slice and serve.

Nutrition info per serving: calories 370, fat 14.3, fiber 3, carbs 14.4, protein 5.6

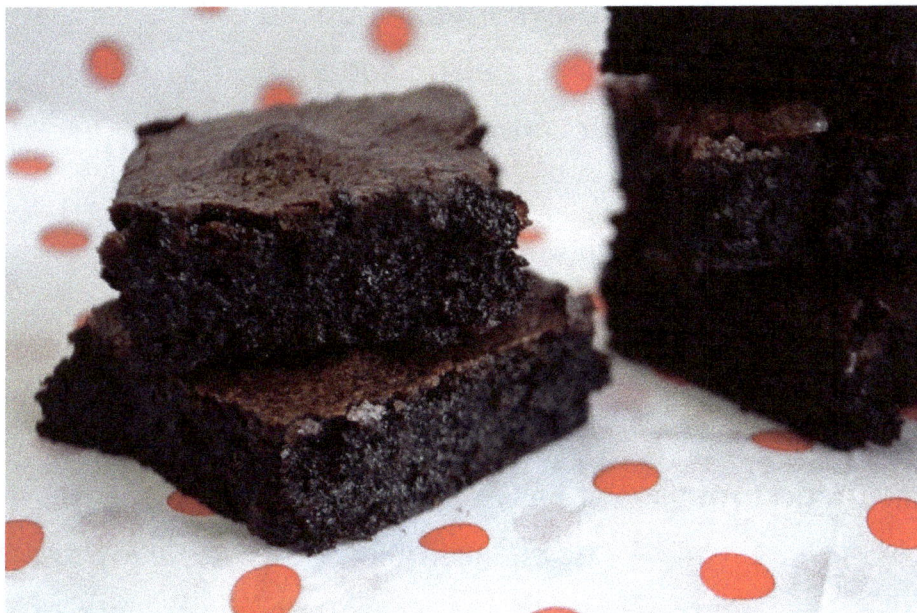

Strawberries Coconut Cake

Prep time: 10 minutes I **Cooking time:** 25 minutes I
Servings: 6

Ingredients:

- 2 cups almond flour
- 1 cup strawberries, chopped
- ½ teaspoon baking soda
- ½ cup coconut sugar
- ¾ cup coconut milk
- ¼ cup avocado oil
- 2 eggs, whisked
- 1 teaspoon vanilla extract
- Cooking spray

Directions:

1. In a bowl, combine the flour with the strawberries and the other ingredients except the coking spray and whisk well.
2. Grease a cake pan with cooking spray, pour the cake mix, spread, bake in the oven at 350 degrees F for 25 minutes, cool down, slice and serve.

Nutrition info per serving: calories 465, fat 22.1, fiber 4, carbs 18.3, protein 13.4

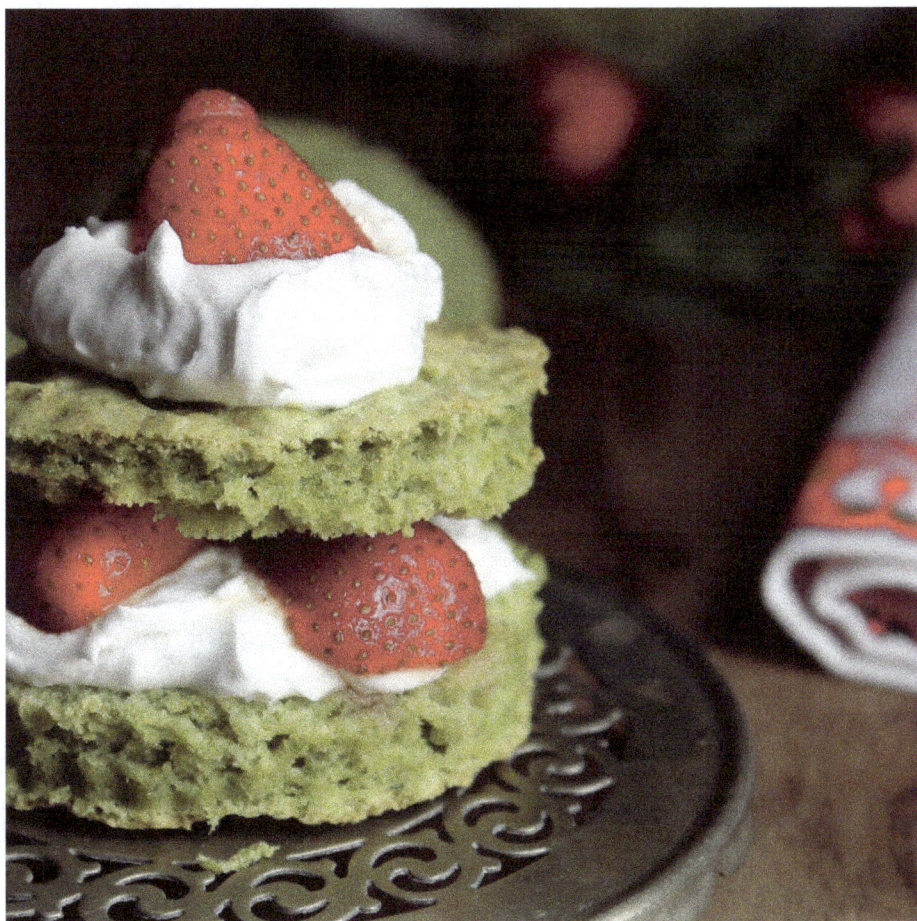

Cocoa Almond Pudding

Prep time: 10 minutes I **Cooking time:** 10 minutes I
Servings: 4

Ingredients:

- 2 tablespoons coconut sugar
- 3 tablespoons coconut flour
- 2 tablespoons cocoa powder
- 2 cups almond milk
- 2 eggs, whisked
- ½ teaspoon vanilla extract

Directions:

1. Put the milk in a pan, add the cocoa and the
   other ingredients, whisk, simmer over medium
   heat for 10 minutes, pour into small cups and
   serve cold.

Nutrition info per serving: calories 385, fat 31.7, fiber
5.7, carbs 21.6, protein 7.3

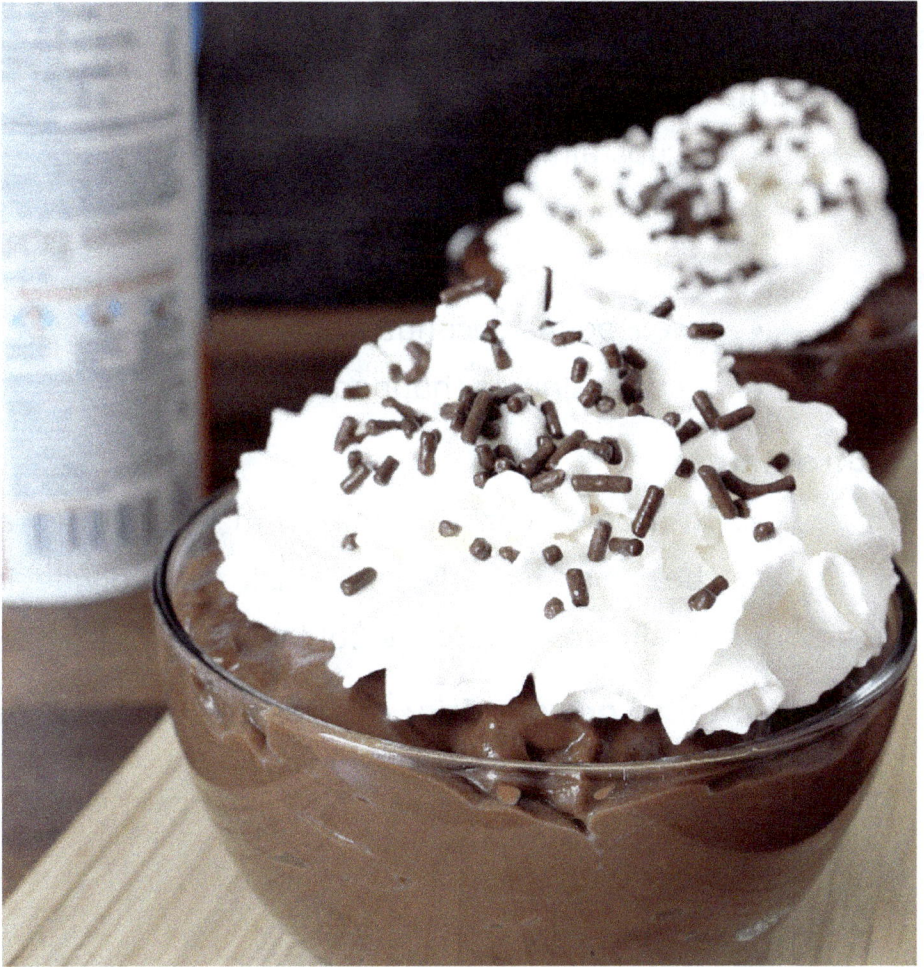

Nutmeg Cream

Prep time: 10 minutes I **Cooking time:** 0 minutes I
Servings: 6

Ingredients:

- 3 cups almond milk
- 1 teaspoon nutmeg, ground
- 2 teaspoons vanilla extract
- 4 teaspoons coconut sugar
- 1 cup walnuts, chopped

Directions:

1. In a bowl, combine milk with the nutmeg and the other ingredients, whisk well, divide into small cups and serve cold.

Nutrition info per serving: calories 243, fat 12.4, fiber 1.5, carbs 21.1, protein 9.7

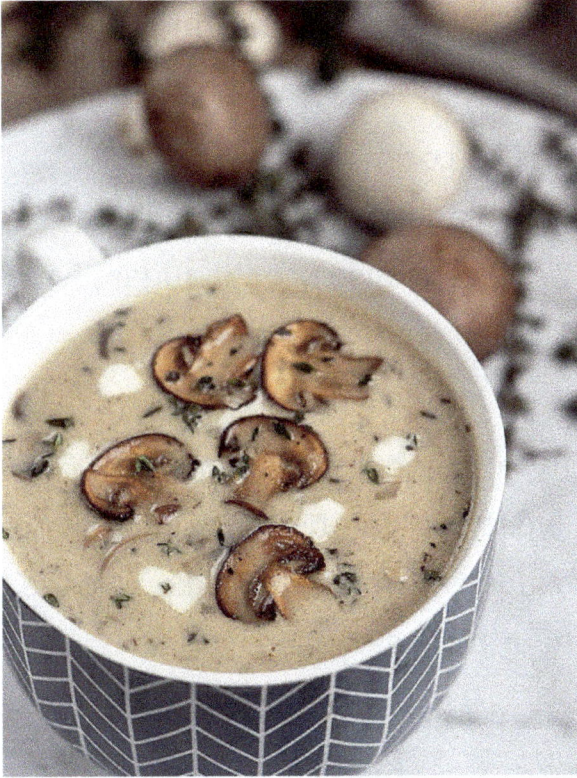

Vanilla Avocado Cream

Prep. time: 1 hour and 10 minutes I **Cooking time:** 0 minutes I **Servings:** 4

Ingredients:

- 2 cups coconut cream
- 2 avocados, peeled, pitted and mashed
- 2 tablespoons coconut sugar
- 1 teaspoon vanilla extract

Directions:

1. In a blender, combine the cream with the avocados and the other ingredients, pulse well, divide into cups and keep in the fridge for 1 hour before serving.

Nutrition info per serving: calories 532, fat 48.2, fiber 9.4, carbs 24.9, protein 5.2

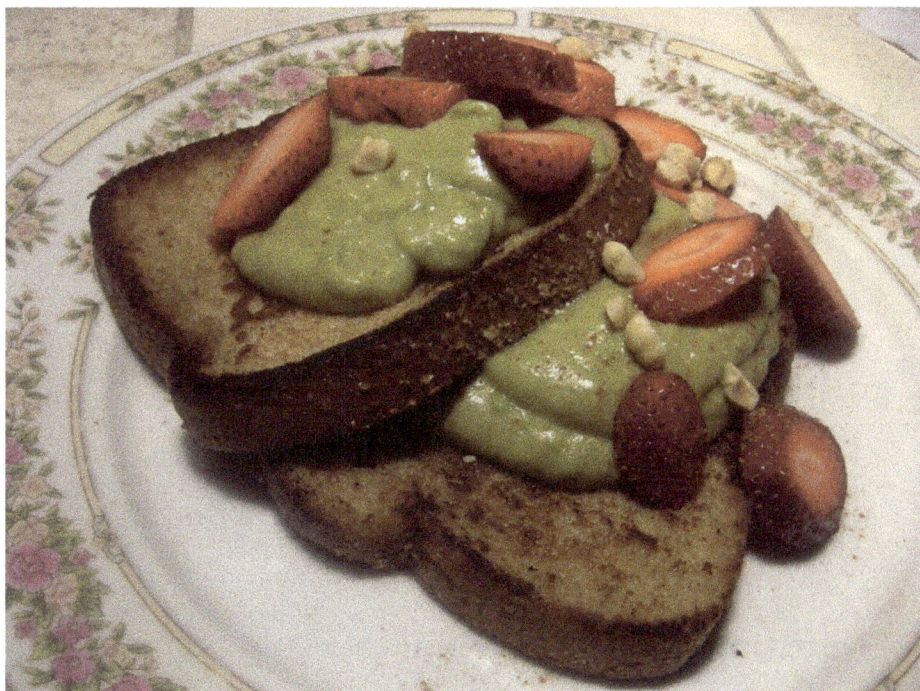

Raspberries Cream Cheese Bowls

Prep time: 10 minutes I **Cooking time:** 25 minutes I
Servings: 4

Ingredients:

- 2 tablespoons almond flour
- 1 cup coconut cream
- 3 cups raspberries
- 1 cup coconut sugar
- 8 ounces cream cheese

Directions:

1. In a bowl, the flour with the cream and the other ingredients, whisk, transfer to a round pan, cook at 360 degrees F for 25 minutes, divide into bowls and serve.

Nutrition info per serving: calories 429, fat 36.3, fiber 7.7, carbs 21.3, protein 7.8

Watermelon Salad

Prep time: 4 minutes I **Cooking time:** 0 minutes I
Servings: 4

Ingredients:

- 1 cup watermelon, peeled and cubed
- 2 apples, cored and cubed
- 1 tablespoon coconut cream
- 2 bananas, cut into chunks

Directions:

1. In a bowl, combine the watermelon with the apples and the other ingredients, toss and serve.

Nutrition info per serving: calories 131, fat 1.3, fiber 4.5, carbs 31.9, protein 1.3

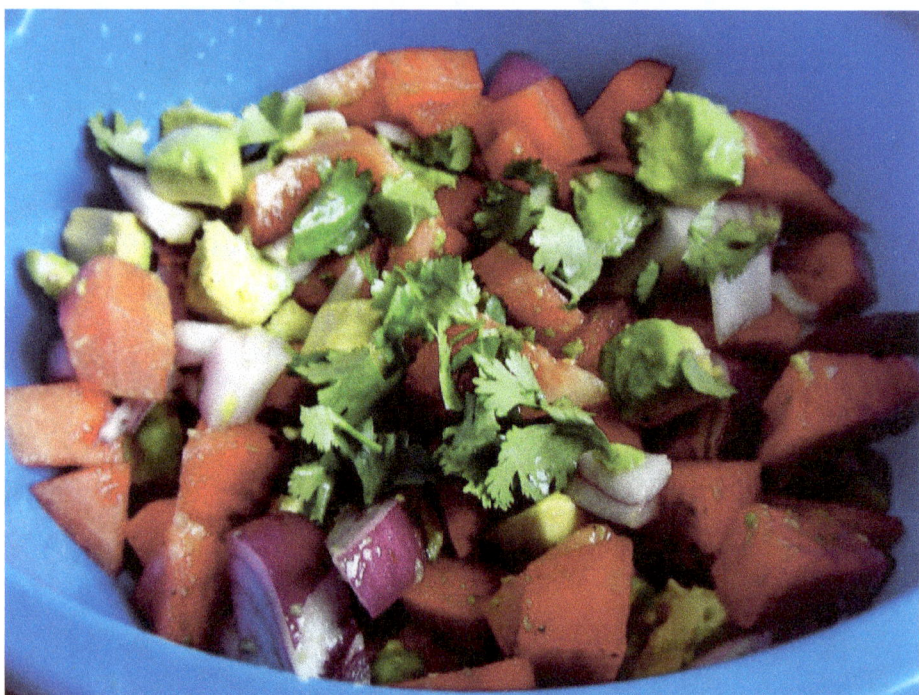

Coconut Apples

Prep time: 10 minutes I **Cooking time:** 10 minutes I **Servings:** 4

Ingredients:

- 2 teaspoons lime juice
- ½ cup coconut cream
- ½ cup coconut, shredded
- 4 apples, cored and cubed
- 4 tablespoons coconut sugar

Directions:

1. In a pan, combine the apples with the lime juice and the other ingredients, stir, bring to a simmer over medium heat and cook for 10 minutes.
2. Divide into bowls and serve cold.

Nutrition info per serving: calories 320, fat 7.8, fiber 3, carbs 6.4, protein 4.7

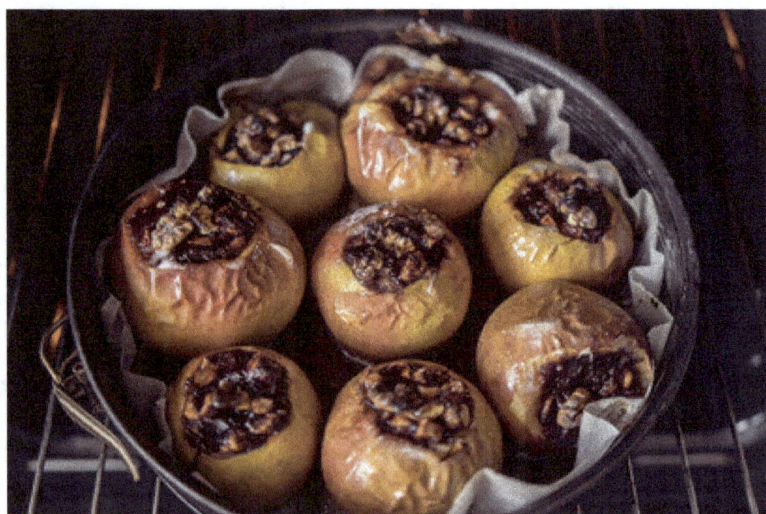

Orange Compote

Prep time: 10 minutes I **Cooking time:** 15 minutes I
Servings: 4

Ingredients:

- 5 tablespoons coconut sugar
- 2 cups orange juice
- 4 oranges, peeled and cut into segments

Directions:

1. In a pot, combine oranges with the sugar and the orange juice, toss, bring to a boil over medium heat, cook for 15 minutes, divide into bowls and serve cold.

Nutrition info per serving: calories 220, fat 5.2, fiber 3, carbs 5.6, protein 5.6

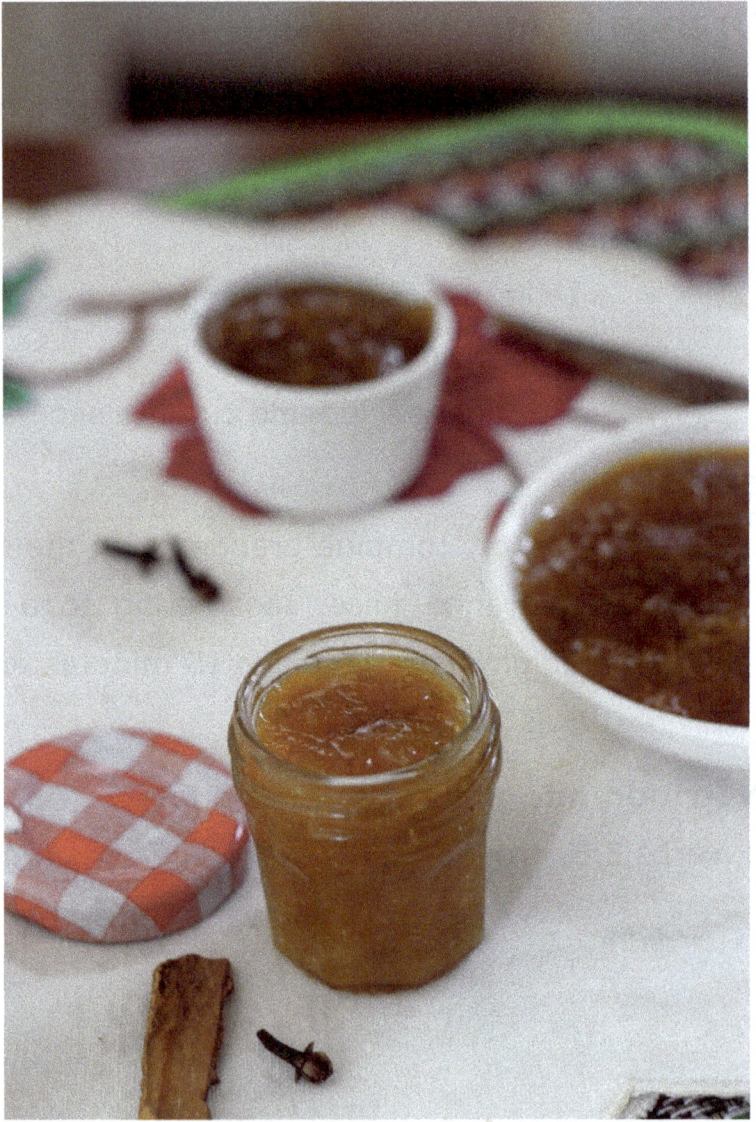

Pears Stew

Prep time: 10 minutes I **Cooking time:** 15 minutes I
Servings: 4

Ingredients:

- 2 cups pears, cored and cut into wedges
- 2 cups water
- 2 tablespoons coconut sugar
- 2 tablespoons lemon juice

Directions:

1. In a pot, combine the pears with the water and the other ingredients, toss, cook over medium heat for 15 minutes, divide into bowls and serve.

Nutrition info per serving: calories 260, fat 6.2, fiber 4.2, carbs 5.6, protein 6

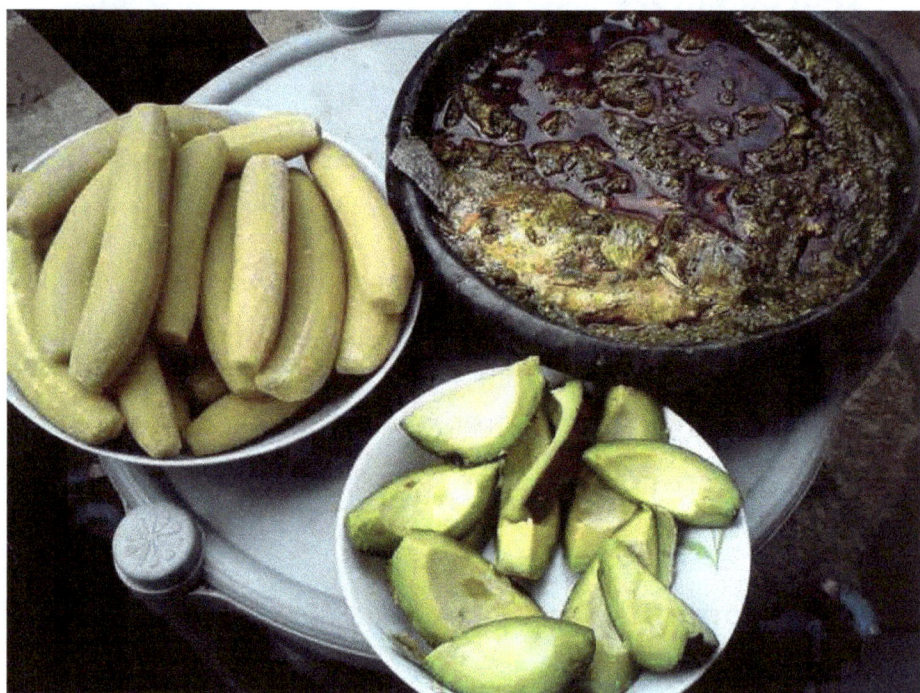

Lemon Watermelon Mix

Prep time: 10 minutes I **Cooking time:** 10 minutes I
Servings: 4

Ingredients:

- 2 cups watermelon, peeled and roughly cubed
- 4 tablespoons coconut sugar
- 2 teaspoons vanilla extract
- 2 teaspoons lemon juice

Directions:

1. In a small pan, combine the watermelon with the sugar and the other ingredients, toss, heat up over medium heat, cook for about 10 minutes, divide into bowls and serve cold.

Nutrition info per serving: calories 140, fat 4, fiber 3.4, carbs 6.7, protein 5

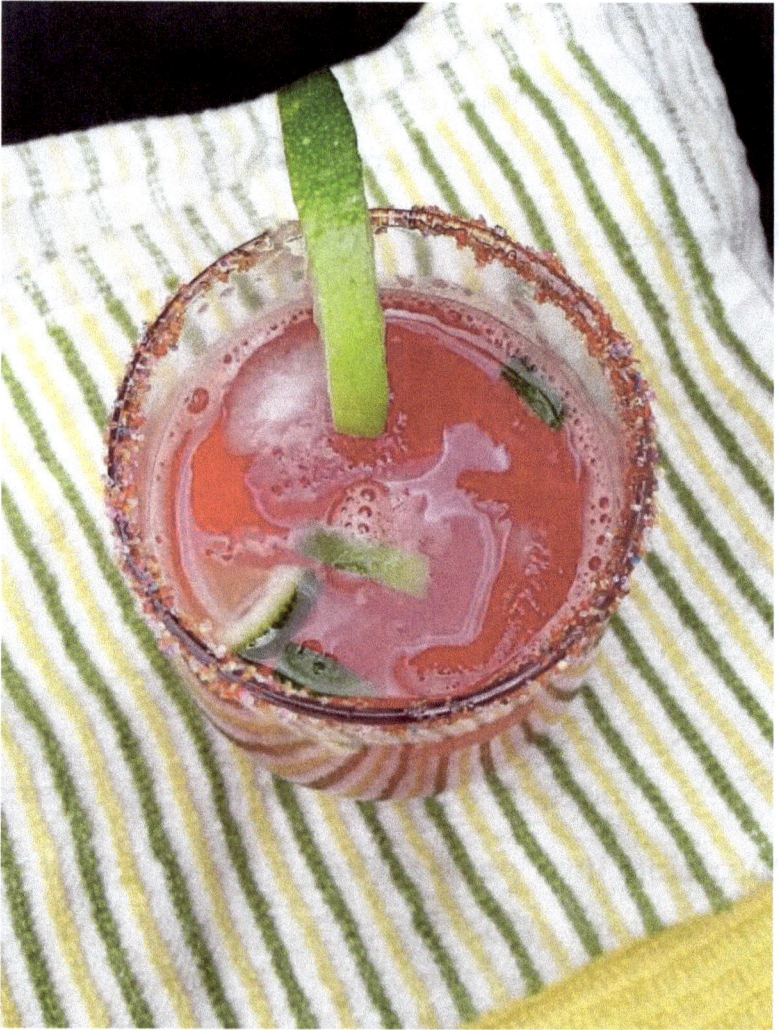

Rhubarb Cream

Prep time: 10 minutes I **Cooking time:** 14 minutes I
Servings: 4

Ingredients:

- 1/3 cup cream cheese
- ½ cup coconut cream
- 2 pound rhubarb, roughly chopped
- 3 tablespoons coconut sugar

Directions:

1. In a blender, combine the cream cheese with the cream and the other ingredients and pulse well.
2. Divide into small cups, introduce in the oven and bake at 350 degrees F for 14 minutes.
3. Serve cold.

Nutrition info per serving: calories 360, fat 14.3, fiber 4.4, carbs 5.8, protein 5.2

Mango Bowls

Prep time: 10 minutes I **Cooking time:** 0 minutes I
Servings: 4

Ingredients:

- 3 cups mango, peeled and cubed
- 1 teaspoon chia seeds
- 1 cup coconut cream
- 1 teaspoon vanilla extract
- 1 tablespoon mint, chopped

Directions:

1. In a bowl, combine the mango with the cream and the other ingredients, toss, divide into smaller bowls and keep in the fridge for 10 minutes before serving.

Nutrition info per serving: calories 238, fat 16.6, fiber 5.6, carbs 22.8, protein 3.3

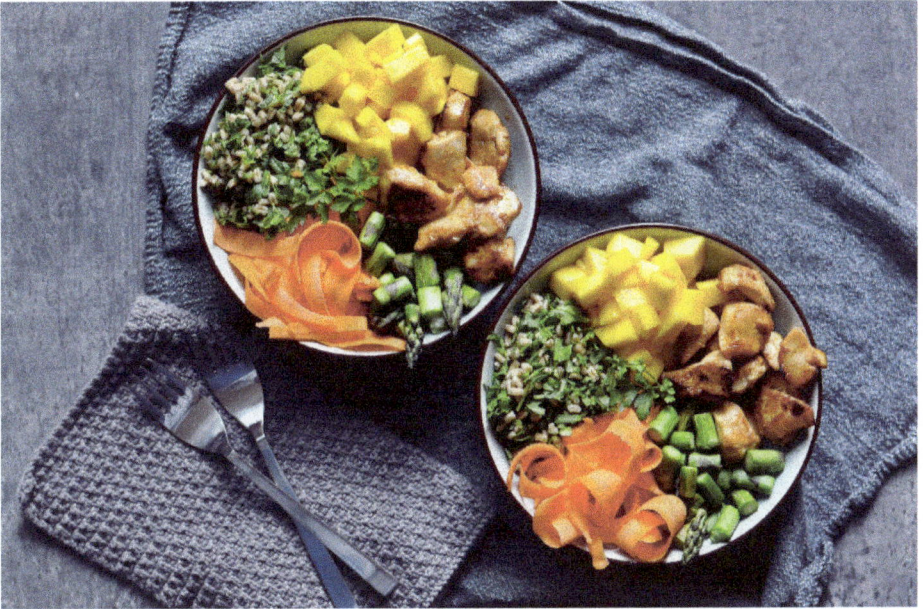

Strawberry Stew

Prep time: 10 minutes I **Cooking time:** 10 minutes I
Servings: 4

Ingredients:

- 2 tablespoons lemon juice
- 1 cup water
- 3 tablespoons coconut sugar
- 12 ounces strawberries, halved

Directions:

1. In a pan, combine the strawberries with the sugar and the other ingredients, bring to a gentle simmer and cook over medium heat for 10 minutes.
2. Divide into bowls and serve.

Nutrition info per serving: calories 122, fat 0.4, fiber 2.1, carbs 26.7, protein 1.5

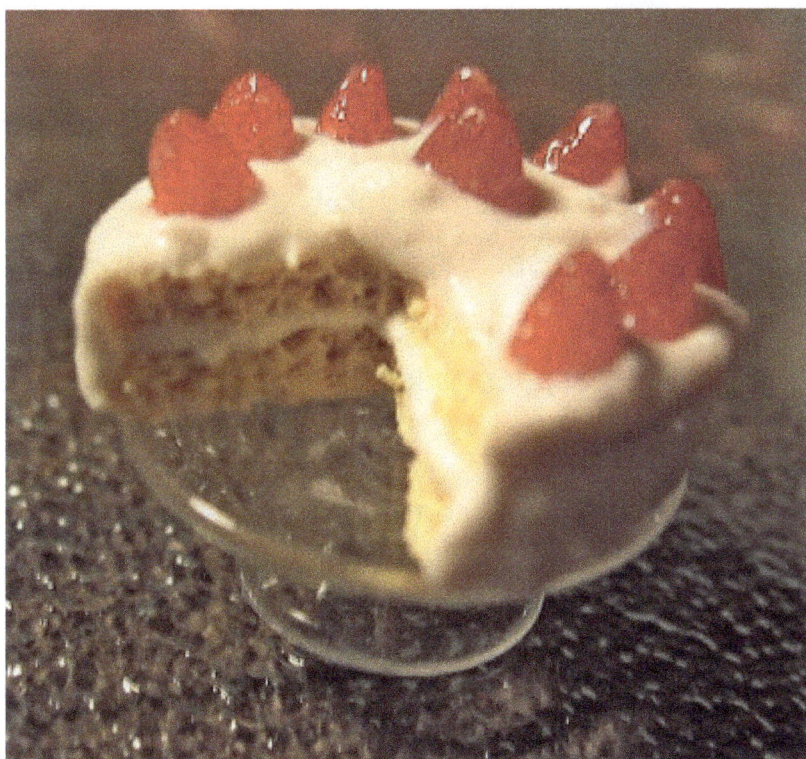

Lemon Pudding

Prep time: 10 minutes I **Cooking time:** 15 minutes I
Servings: 4

Ingredients:

- 2 cups coconut cream
- Juice of 1 lemon
- Zest of 1 lemon, grated
- 3 tablespoons avocado oil
- 1 egg, whisked
- 1 teaspoon baking powder

Directions:

1. In a bowl, combine the cream with the lemon juice and the other ingredients and whisk well.
2. Divide into small ramekins, introduce in the oven and bake at 360 degrees F for 15 minutes.
3. Serve the pudding cold.

Nutrition info per serving: calories 385, fat 39.9, fiber 2.7, carbs 8.2, protein 4.2

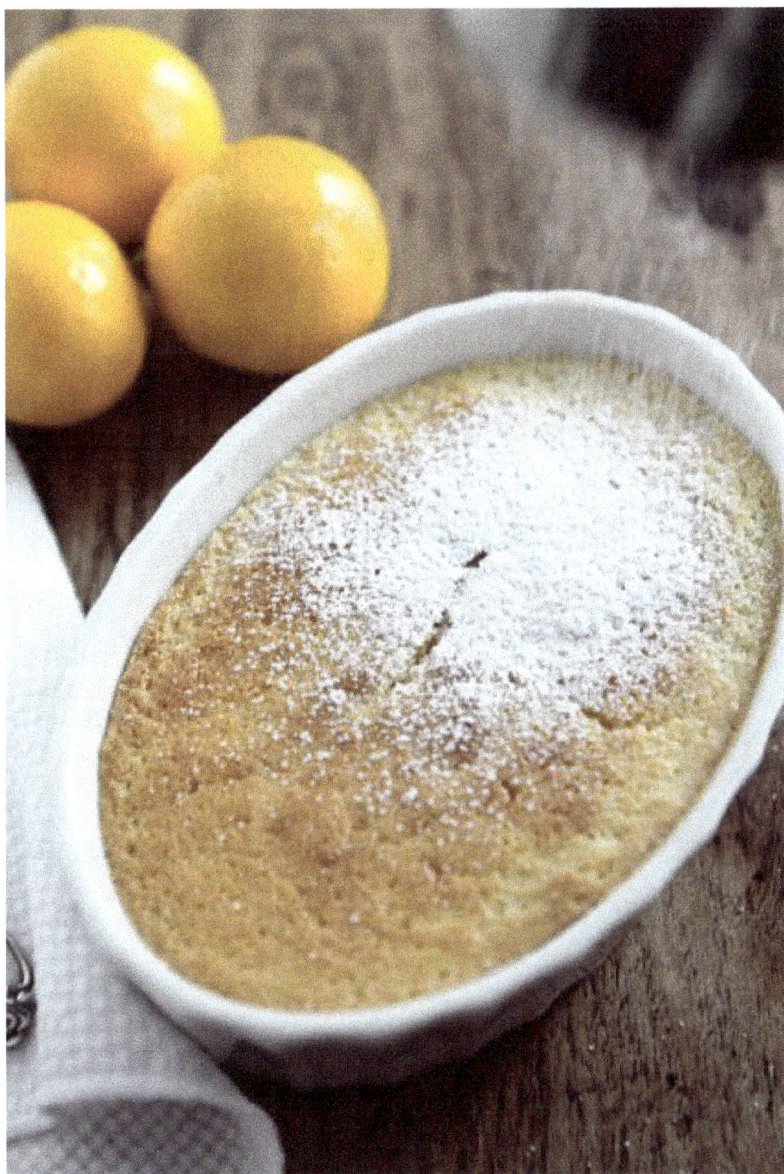

Peach Cream

Prep time: 10 minutes I **Cooking time:** 0 minutes I
Servings: 4

Ingredients:

- 3 cups coconut cream
- 2 peaches, stones removed and chopped
- 1 teaspoon vanilla extract
- ½ cup almonds, chopped

Directions:

1. In a blender, combine the cream and the other ingredients, pulse well, divide into small bowls and serve cold.

Nutrition info per serving: calories 261, fat 13, fiber 5.6, carbs 7, protein 5.4

Vanilla Plums

Prep time: 10 minutes I **Cooking time:** 15 minutes I
Servings: 4

Ingredients:

- 1 pound plums, stones removed and halved
- 2 tablespoons coconut sugar
- ½ teaspoon vanilla extract
- 1 cup water

Directions:

1. In a pan, combine the plums with the sugar and the other ingredients, bring to a simmer and cook over medium heat for 15 minutes.
2. Divide into bowls and serve cold.

Nutrition info per serving: calories 142, fat 4, fiber 2.4, carbs 14, protein 7

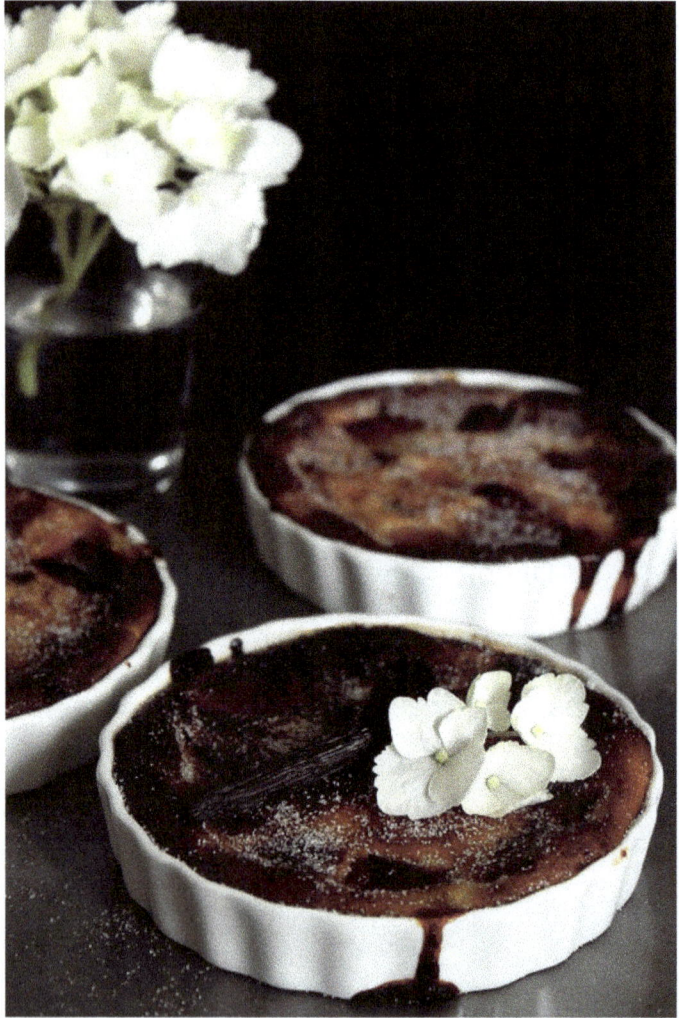

Chia Apples

Prep time: 10 minutes I **Cooking time:** 10 minutes I **Servings:** 4

Ingredients:

- 2 cups apples, cored and cut into wedges
- 2 tablespoons chia seeds
- 1 teaspoon vanilla extract
- 2 cups naturally unsweetened apple juice

Directions:

1. In a small pot, combine the apples with the chia seeds and the other ingredients, toss, cook over medium heat for 10 minutes, divide into bowls and serve cold.

Nutrition info per serving: calories 172, fat 5.6, fiber 3.5, carbs 10, protein 4.4

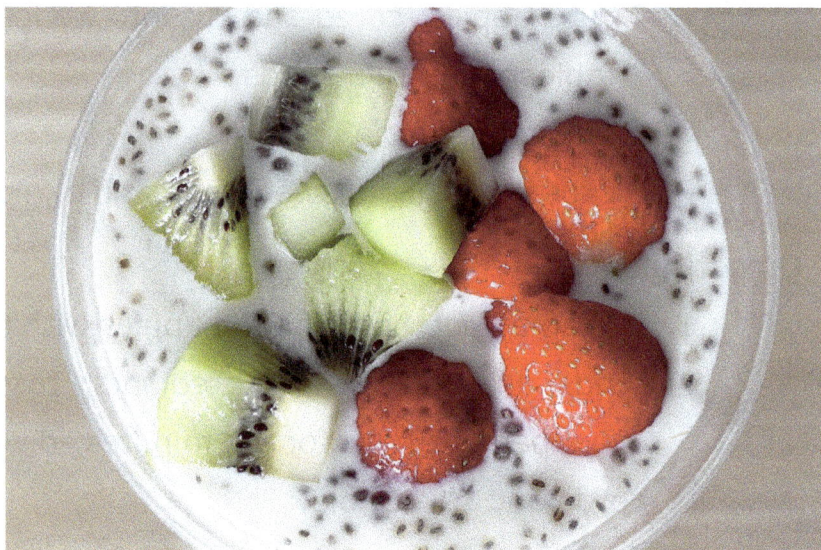

Rice Pudding

Prep time: 10 minutes I **Cooking time:** 25 minutes I
Servings: 4

Ingredients:

- 6 cups water
- 1 cup coconut sugar
- 2 cups black rice
- 2 pears, cored and cubed
- 2 teaspoons cinnamon powder

Directions:

1. Put the water in a pan, heat it up over medium-high heat, add the rice, sugar and the other ingredients, stir, bring to a simmer, reduce heat to medium and cook for 25 minutes.
2. Divide into bowls and serve cold.

Nutrition info per serving: calories 290, fat 13.4, fiber 4, carbs 13.20, protein 6.7

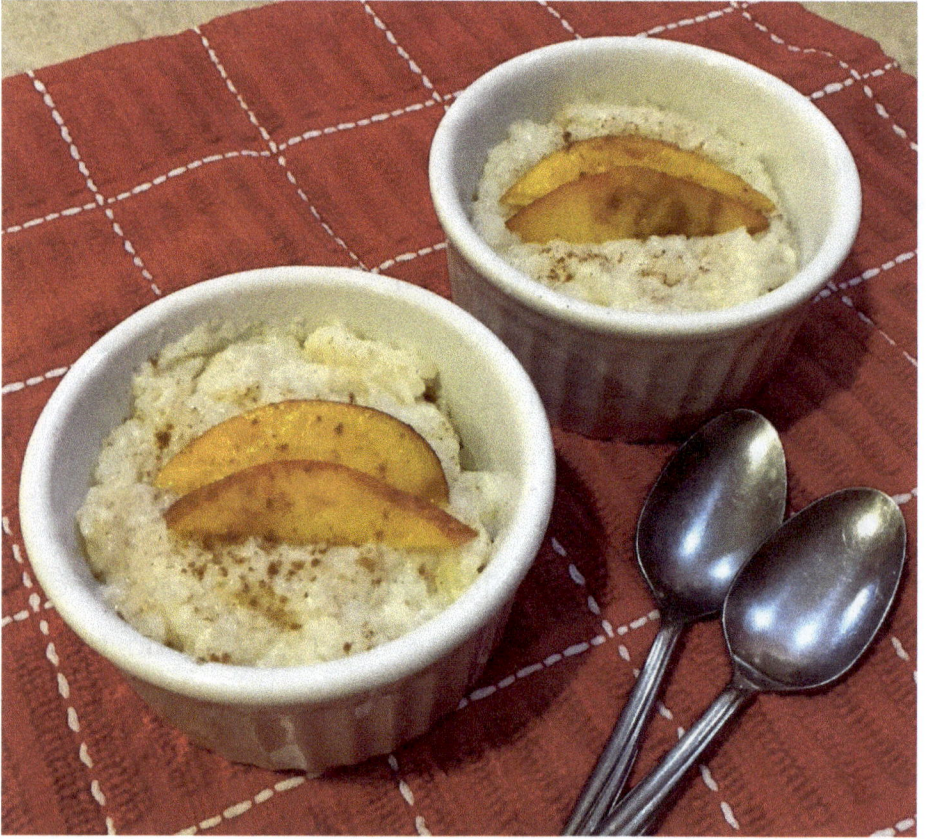

Almond Rhubarb Bowls

Prep time: 10 minutes I **Cooking time:** 15 minutes I
Servings: 4

Ingredients:

- 2 cups rhubarb, roughly chopped
- 3 tablespoons coconut sugar
- 1 teaspoon almond extract
- 2 cups water

Directions:

1. In a pot, combine the rhubarb with the other ingredients, toss, bring to a boil over medium heat, cook for 15 minutes, divide into bowls and serve cold.

Nutrition info per serving: calories 142, fat 4.1, fiber 4.2, carbs 7, protein 4

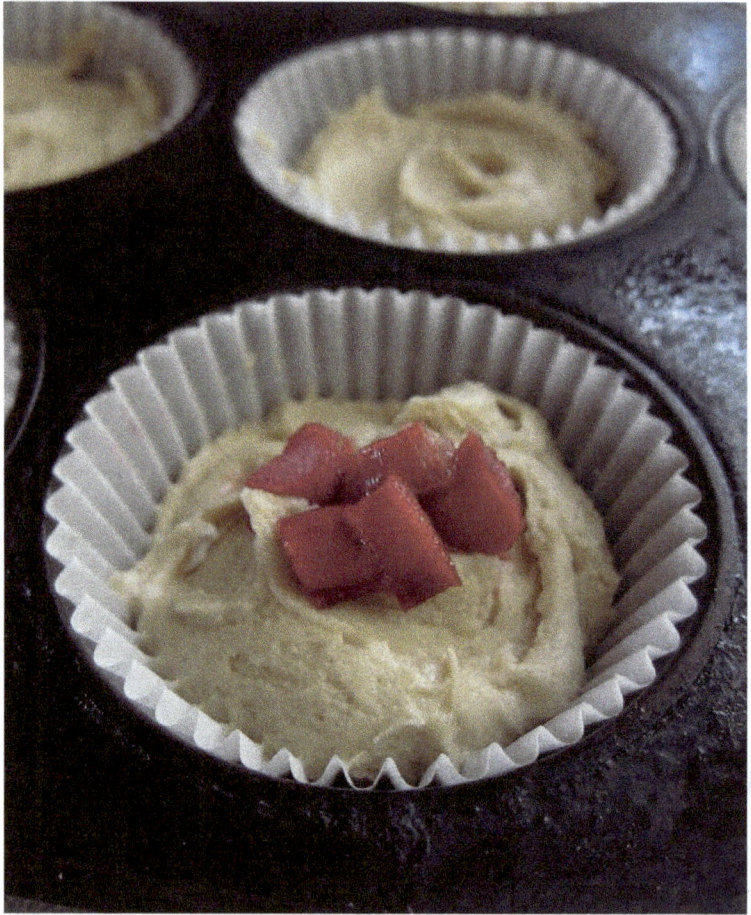

Lime Berry Cream

Prep time: 1 hour I **Cooking time:** 10 minutes I
Servings: 4

Ingredients:

- 2 cups coconut cream
- 1 cup blueberries
- 3 eggs, whisked
- 3 tablespoons coconut sugar
- 1 tablespoon lime juice

Directions:

1. In a small pan, combine the cream with the berries and the other ingredients, whisk well, simmer over medium heat for 10 minutes, blend using an immersion blender, divide into bowls and keep in the fridge for 1 hour before serving.

Nutrition info per serving: calories 230, fat 8.4, fiber 2.4, carbs 7.8, protein 6

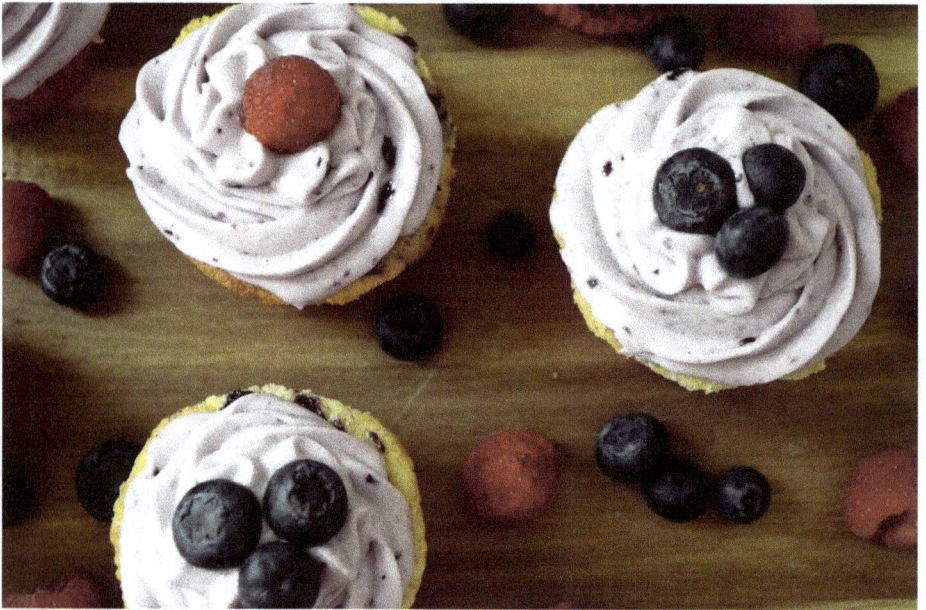

Mint Blueberries Bowls

Prep time: 5 minutes I **Cooking time:** 0 minutes I
Servings: 4

Ingredients:

- 2 cups blueberries
- 3 tablespoons mint, chopped
- 1 pear, cored and cubed
- 1 apple, core and cubed
- 1 tablespoon coconut sugar

Directions:

1. In a bowl, combine the blueberries with the mint and the other ingredients, toss and serve cold.

Nutrition info per serving: calories 150, fat 2.4, fiber 4, carbs 6.8, protein 6

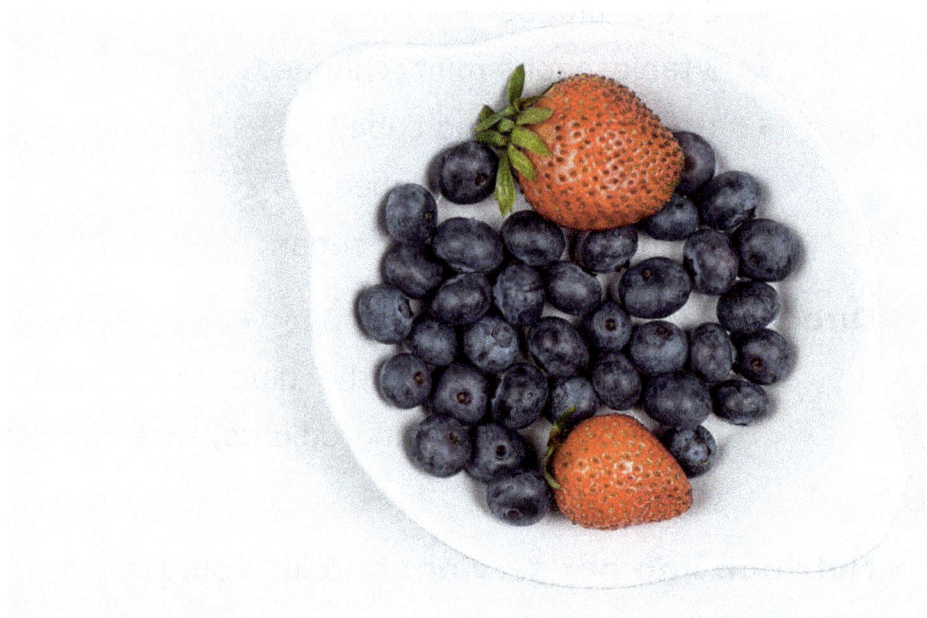

Banana Cream

Prep time: 5 minutes I **Cooking time:** 0 minutes I

Servings: 4

Ingredients:

- 1 cup almond milk
- 1 banana, peeled and sliced
- 1 teaspoon vanilla extract
- ½ cup coconut cream
- dates, chopped

Directions:

1. In a blender, combine the dates with the banana and the other ingredients, pulse well, divide into small cups and serve cold.

Nutrition info per serving: calories 271, fat 21.6, fiber 3.8, carbs 21.2, protein 2.7

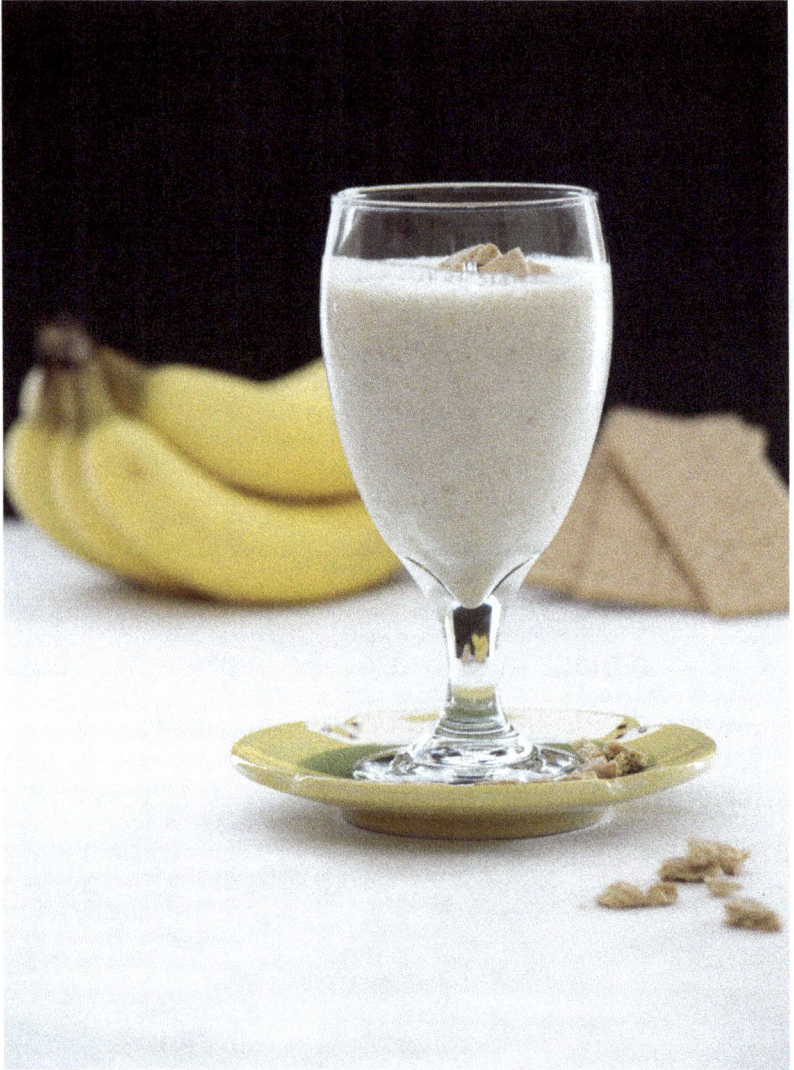

Muffins

Prep time: 10 minutes I **Cooking time:** 25 minutes I
Servings: 12

Ingredients:

- 3 tablespoons avocado oil
- ½ cup almond milk
- 4 eggs, whisked
- 1 teaspoon vanilla extract
- 1 cup almond flour
- 2 teaspoons cinnamon powder
- ½ teaspoon baking powder
- 1 cup plums, pitted and chopped

Directions:

1. In a bowl, combine the oil with the almond milk and the other ingredients and whisk well.
2. Divide into a muffin pan, introduce in the oven at 350 degrees F and bake for 25 minutes.
3. Serve the muffins cold.

Nutrition info per serving: calories 270, fat 3.4, fiber 4.4, carbs 12, protein 5

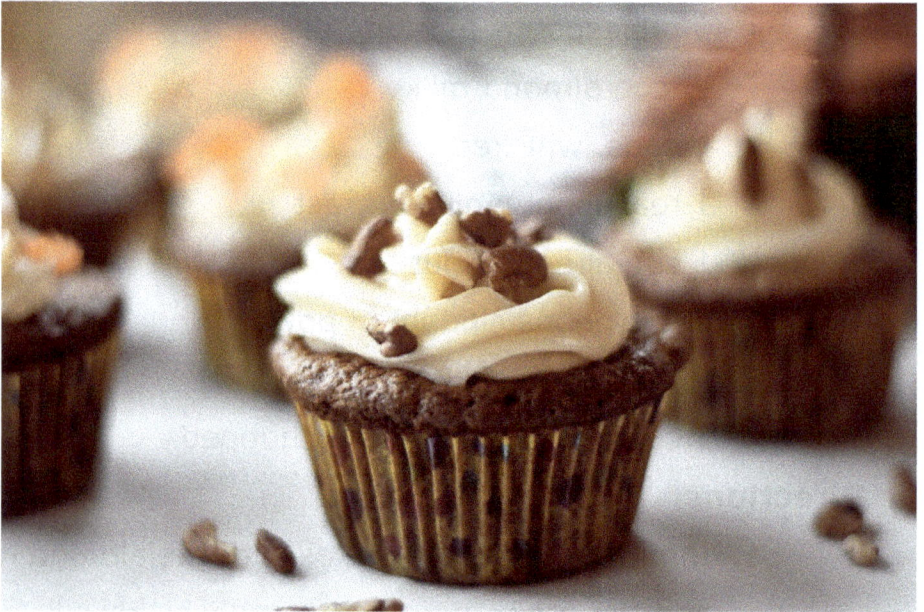

Plums Bowls

Prep time: 10 minutes I **Cooking time:** 20 minutes I
Servings: 4

Ingredients:

- ½ pound plums, pitted and halved
- 2 tablespoons coconut sugar
- 4 tablespoons raisins
- 1 teaspoon vanilla extract
- 1 cup coconut cream

Directions:

1. In a pan, combine the plums with the sugar and the other ingredients, bring to a simmer and cook over medium heat for 20 minutes.
2. Divide into bowls and serve.

Nutrition info per serving: calories 219, fat 14.4, fiber 1.8, carbs 21.1, protein 2.2

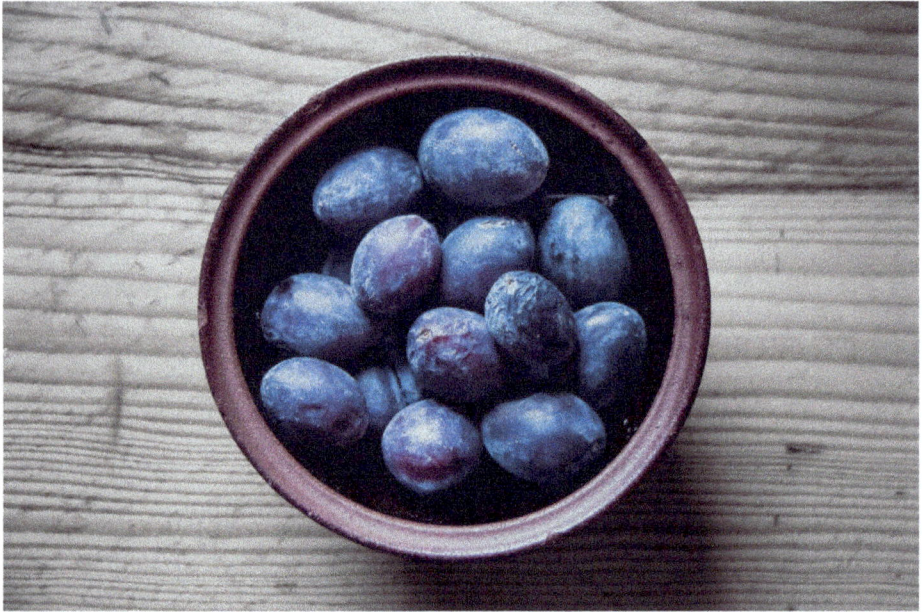

Seed Bars

Prep time: 10 minutes I **Cooking time:** 20 minutes I
Servings: 6

Ingredients:

- 1 cup coconut flour
- ½ teaspoon baking soda
- 1 tablespoon flax seed
- 3 tablespoons almond milk
- 1 cup sunflower seeds
- 2 tablespoons coconut oil, melted
- 1 teaspoon vanilla extract

Directions:

1. In a bowl, mix the flour with the baking soda and the other ingredients, stir really well, spread on a baking sheet, press well, bake in the oven at 350 degrees F for 20 minutes, leave aside to cool down, cut into bars and serve.

Nutrition info per serving: calories 189, fat 12.6, fiber 9.2, carbs 15.7, protein 4.7

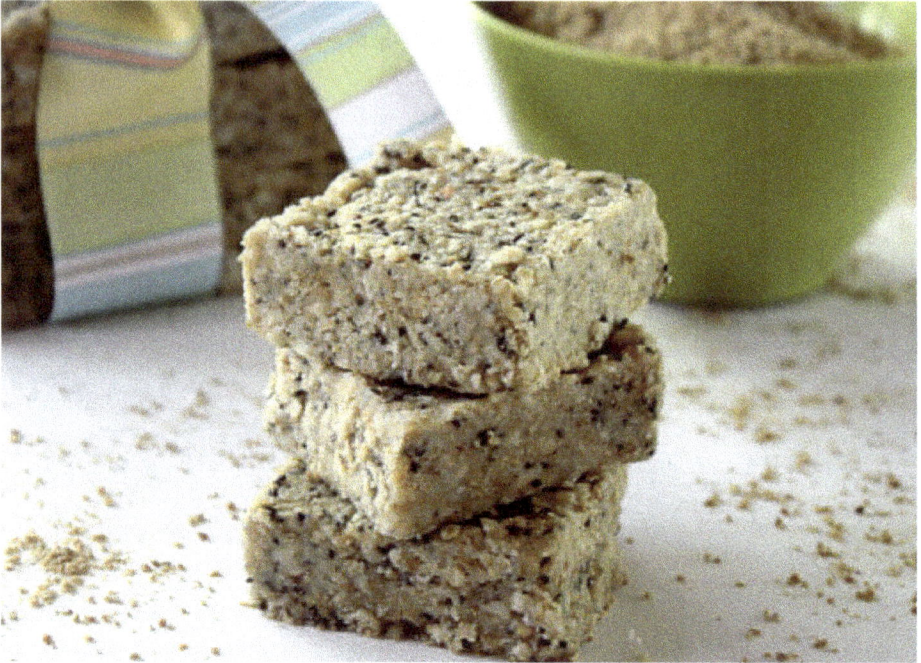

www.ingramcontent.com/pod-product-compliance
Lightning Source LLC
Chambersburg PA
CBHW050754030426
42336CB00012B/1818